The Environment and Social Policy

This introductory text focuses on human welfare and the environment from a social policy perspective. It shows how environmental concerns are becoming increasingly central to social policy and discusses the roles of central and local government in relation to environmental issues.

The Environment and Social Policy covers the following contemporary topics:

- sustainability
- Local Agenda 21
- green ideas
- environmental health
- housing and urban development
- food
- work
- globalisation.

Each chapter starts with an overview of the topic and ends with a list of key points and a guide to further reading. Core concepts are clearly explained and illustrated throughout this text, which provides students with a concise and up-to-date summary of what they need to know.

Michael Cahill is Reader in Social Policy at the University of Brighton.

The Gildredge Social Policy Series

The Gildredge Social Policy Series provides introductory textbooks to key areas of policy for the growing number of students of social policy at A level, A/S level, on GNVQ courses, in their first year at university, or following a professional diploma course. Written by experienced teachers, the books are short, tightly structured texts designed to be aids to learning.

Series editor: **Pete Alcock**, Professor of Social Policy and Administration, the University of Birmingham.

Also in the series

Education Policy	Paul Trowler
Crime and Social Policy	Mike Stephens
Social Work and Social Care	Lester Parrott
Family Policy	Fran Wasoff and Ian Dey
Health Policy	Ann Wall and Barry Owen
Housing Policy	Jean Conway

The Environment
and Social Policy

Michael Cahill

London and New York

HN
17.5
.C3
2002

4681'2053

First published 2002
by Routledge
11 New Fetter Lane, London EC4P 4EE

Simultaneously published in the USA and Canada
by Routledge
29 West 35th Street, New York, NY 10001

Routledge is an imprint of the Taylor & Francis Group

Typeset in Times by
Prepress Projects Ltd, Perth, Scotland
Printed and bound in Great Britain by
TJ International Ltd, Padstow, Cornwall

British Library Cataloguing in Publication Data
A catalogue record for this book is available
from the British Library

Library of Congress Cataloging in Publication Data
Cahill, Michael, 1951–
    The environment and social policy / Michael Cahill.
        p. cm. (Gildredge social policy series)
    Includes bibliographical references and index.
    ISBN 0-415-26105-8 (hbk) – ISBN 0-953-35718-X (pbk)
    1. Social policy – Environmental aspects. 2. Environmental policy.
    3. Environmental protection. 4. Sustainable development. I. Title II. Series.

HC17.5 .C3 2001
361.6'–dc21   2001019936

To my mother and the memory of my father

Contents

Illustrations   viii
Acknowledgements   x

1   Sustainability and social policy   1

2   Sustainable development   19

3   Local Agenda 21   30

4   Green ideas   47

5   Environmental health   65

6   Housing and urban development   92

7   Food   113

8   Work   133

9   One world   153

Bibliography   168
Index   177

Illustrations

Boxes

1.1	The Brundtland Report	5
2.1	The Fifth EU Environmental Action Programme	24
2.2	Government's headline indicators	27
3.1	The Local Agenda 21 process	34
4.1	'The Tragedy of the Commons'	54
4.2	The eight basic principles of deep ecology	56
5.1	Main effects of global climate change on population health	66
5.2	The adverse health effects of air pollution	72
5.3	Health hazards from transport pollutants	74
5.4	World Health Organization action plan for member states on transport, environment and health	76
7.1	Organic food	117
7.2	The role of the Food Standards Agency	130
9.1	The global context	155

Figures

6.1	Population change in the urban areas of England 1961–94	100
6.2	Room temperature and associated risks	107

Tables

3.1   Stakeholder groups   38
5.1   Transport accidents, 1977, 1987 and 1994   78
5.2   Noise sources outside dwellings, 1986–91   80
5.3   Factors affecting health   85
6.1   The effect of policy initiatives on the fuel poor
      and environmental pollution   108
7.1   Children's food consumption, 1950 and 1993   123
7.2   Food poisoning   127
7.3   Genetically modified food   128
8.1   Potential of LETS to re-engage individuals
      into the local economy   147
9.1   Top corporations and their sales compared
      with the gross domestic product (GDP) of selected
      countries in 1997   156
9.2   Ecological footprints of leading industrial nations   162

Acknowledgements

My thanks to Pete Alcock for suggesting that I write this book and to Patrick McNeill for his editorial suggestions, which greatly improved the text. The book is a much better one because of the careful reading that Meg Huby afforded it and I am grateful to her for this assistance. Thanks are also extended to the following, who read parts of the text and gave me the benefit of their critical comments: John Baker, John Davies, Ian McHugh, Bob Skelton and Marilyn Taylor. As ever, I am indebted to Vanessa, Thomas and Grace for their love and support. In a book of this kind, which draws upon a mass of published material, there will inevitably be some errors and I apologise for these in advance.

Michael Cahill
August 2001

Copyright acknowledgements

Box 1.1 has been reproduced from the Brundtland Report (1987) *Our Common Future*, with permission from Oxford University Press.

Box 2.2 has been reproduced from Department of the Environment, Transport and the Regions (1999) *A Better Quality of Life: a Strategy for Sustainable Development in the UK*, Cm. 4345, Crown copyright, and is reproduced with the permission of the Controller of Her Majesty's Stationery Office.

Table 3.1 has been adapted from Freeman, C., Littlewood, S. and Whitney, D. (1996) 'Local government and emerging models of participation in the Local Agenda 21 process', *Journal of Environmental Planning and Management* 39, 65–78. See the journal's web site at http://www.tandf.co.uk.

Box 4.1 has been reprinted with permission from Hardin, G. (1968) in Daly, H.E. (ed.) (1980) *Economics, Ecology, Ethics, Essays Towards a Steady-state Economy*, San Francisco: W. H. Freeman. Copyright 1980 American Association for the Advancement of Science.

Box 4.2 has been reprinted from Devall and Sessions in Pepper, D. (1996) *Modern Environmentalism, an Introduction*, with permission from Routledge.

Box 5.1 has been reprinted from McMichael, A.J. (1993) *Planetary Overload, Global Environmental Change and the Health of the Human Species*, with permission from Cambridge University Press.

Box 5.3 has been reprinted from Potter, S. (1997) *Vital Travel Statistics* with permission from Landor Publishing.

Table 5.1 has been reprinted from Potter, S. (1997) *Vital Travel Statistics* with permission from Landor Publishing.

Table 5.2 has been reprinted from Maddison, D. *et al.* (1996) *The True Costs of Road Transport* with permission from Kogan Page.

Table 5.3 has been reprinted from Department of Health (1998a) *Our Healthier Nation, a Contract for Health*, Cm. 3852, Crown copyright, and is reproduced with the permission of the Controller of Her Majesty's Stationery Office.

Figure 6.1 has been reprinted from the Office for National Statistics Regional Trends (1992), Crown copyright, and is reproduced with the permission of the Controller of Her Majesty's Stationery Office.

Figure 6.2 has been reprinted from Department of the Environment, Transport and the Regions (1999) *Fuel Poverty, The New HEES*, London: DETR, Crown copyright, and is reproduced with the permission of the Controller of Her Majesty's Stationery Office.

Table 6.1 has been reprinted from Carley, M. and Kirk, K. (1998)

Sustainable by 2020? with permission from The Policy Press and the Joseph Rowntree Foundation.

Table 6.2 has been reprinted from Bhatti, M., Brooke, J. and Gibson, M. (eds) (1994) *Housing and the Environment; a New Agenda* with permission from the Chartered Institute of Housing.

Table 7.1 has been reprinted with permission from Meikle, J. (1999) 'Children's diet healthier in 1950 than today', *Guardian* 30 November.

Table 7.2 has been reprinted with permission from Meikle, J. (1998) 'Food poisoning', *Guardian* 14 January.

Table 8.1 has been reprinted from Hudson, H., Newby, L., Hutchinson, N. with Harding, L. (1999) *Making 'LETS' Work in Low Income Areas* with permission from Forum for the Future.

Table 9.2 has been reprinted from Mayo, E. (1998) *Making New Economics, Proposals for the G8 1998 Summits* with permission from the New Economics Foundation.

Chapter 1
Sustainability and social policy

Outline

Industrialisation brought untold wealth and transformed the way of life of the populations of the rich world in the nineteenth century, but it also produced social problems: poor housing, ill-health and poverty. Government intervention in the form of social policies was aimed at alleviating these social problems. Industrialisation and urbanisation, which by the late twentieth century had become a global phenomenon, resulted in serious environmental problems: resource depletion, climate change and widespread pollution. Consumer societies have exacerbated the environmental problems through their large-scale use of natural resources, their polluting processes and the transport infrastructures that they have created. The reaction to the developing environmental crisis has been widespread and has taken a variety of forms. This chapter focuses on the concept of sustainability because it has dominated environmental politics, and also considers the connections among consumer societies, the environmental agenda and social policy. It also examines the ways in which the environmental debate has linked with the debate on social inequality.

Sustainability

Sustainability is a 'hurrah word' in contemporary political debate – everyone is in favour of it just as we are all in favour of democracy or justice. The government has taken to spraying the word all over many of its policy papers and reports: sustainable transport policy, sustainable housing, sustainable health care. Sustainability and sustainable development are often used interchangeably, and they are at times used in this way in this book, but the two terms need to be distinguished: sustainability is the end-state, whereas sustainable development is the means to achieving that end. Sustainable development has been best defined as development which 'meets the needs of the present, without compromising the ability of future generations to meet their own needs' (Brundtland Report, 1987: 8). Sustainability and sustainable development are ambitious concepts for they integrate environmental, economic and social policy. This book is about the 'how to' policies which would enable a sustainable society to emerge, and so it is concerned with 'sustainable development' in social policy. Jacobs has identified six core themes in the contemporary debate on sustainability. These are:

- integration of environmental considerations in economic planning;
- futurity: concern about the impact of contemporary decisions on future generations;
- environmental protection: policies to reduce environmental damage;
- equity: commitment to meeting the basic needs of the poor today and in the future;
- quality of life: economic growth does not equate with human well-being;
- participation: sustainable development requires as much involvement as possible by individuals and groups if it is to work (Jacobs in Dobson, 1999: 26–7).

Social policy

Social policy is concerned with the satisfaction of human needs – for shelter, for food, etc. – for those people whose needs cannot be met by the working of the economic system because they are perhaps too poor, too old or too young or they are too disabled to work. The meeting of need has an environmental impact: how we produce food, organise housing and look after our health-care needs, for example, have environmental consequences and will affect future generations.

Social policy is central to discussions of sustainability because it is a major means by which governments provide a minimum level of support for the population. It has been a central feature of government policies in the rich world since 1945. Although the administrative and organisational arrangements differ widely, the 'welfare state' has been a component of government policy in most developed countries. The welfare state provides income maintenance, education, housing, health care and social services. Welfare states have been one of the achievements of most industrial societies, but these services are not immune from environmental considerations – they have an impact on the environment through their buildings, policies and the activities of their work force. Social policy can be used to reduce inequalities within society, and there is a variety of ways in which this can be done, e.g. by taxation which redistributes wealth or by spending programmes which benefit those living in poor areas. It could also involve the reduction of inequalities which result from the impact of environmental pollution. Social policy emerged in the nineteenth century as a response to the social problems produced by the impact of humanity on the environment. This is explored in the next section.

Industrialisation and the environment

The natural environment is the basis upon which human life and achievements are built – we cannot exist apart from it, and until the second half of the twentieth century nature was the dominant partner in the relationship between human beings and nature. Since the onset of industrialisation in the middle of the eighteenth century in Britain, humankind has been utilising natural resources – coal, water, minerals – at an accelerating rate. Social policy was a reaction to the social problems produced by the twin pressures of industrial processes and urbanisation. A great many of these social problems were related to the environmental damage produced by industrialisation and urbanisation: rivers were polluted by factories and became a health hazard and the dumping of industrial waste into streams had the result of contaminating clean water supplies.

Atmospheric pollution was widespread in industrial areas from the coal used by furnaces, railway engines and gasworks. Coal was the major source of domestic heating and energy and thus added to the pollution.

After 1945 industrialisation and urbanisation steadily became global realities and the pressures on the environment increased substantially. We have now reached the point at which nature has been profoundly affected by the enterprise of human beings, and in our time nature is now responding to the stress and despoliation it has suffered. Nature is delicately balanced with complex inter-relationships between species. The growing power of humanity and the way in which humans have regarded nature as seemingly an inexhaustible source of resources for human activity has changed the balance between humans and nature. Atomic weaponry meant that since the 1940s human beings have had the means to destroy nature over a wide area and indeed, if used, the present stock of nuclear devices could destroy the world many times over. The burning of fossil fuels and the clearing of forests which have contributed to global warming are the results of this indifference to the impact of human activity on nature. The result of industrialisation and the pressure of human population has been widespread environmental damage, and this has accelerated in recent years.

Brundtland Report

The contemporary usage of the concept of sustainability can be traced back to the report of the international commission headed by Gro Brundtland, a former Norwegian Prime Minister, which examined the relationship between development and environmental issues. The report defines sustainable development as 'development that meets the needs of the present without compromising the ability of future generations to meet their own needs' (Brundtland Report, 1987: 43) (Box 1.1). Pointing out that the essential needs of millions of people – for shelter, for food, for jobs – were not being met, the report proposed economic growth which did not endanger the planet's life-support systems of water, soil and the atmosphere. The report was the first major document which combined the

Box 1.1 The Brundtland Report

Sustainable development

Humanity has the ability to make development sustainable – to ensure that it meets the needs of the present without compromising the ability of future generations to meet their own needs. The concept of sustainable development does imply limits – not absolute limits but limitations imposed by the present state of technology and social organisation on environmental resources and by the ability of the biosphere to absorb the effects of human activities. But technology and social organisation can be both managed and improved to make way for a new era of economic growth. The Commission believes that widespread poverty is no longer inevitable. Poverty is not only an evil in itself, but sustainable development requires meeting the basic needs of all and the extending to all the opportunity to fulfil their aspirations for a better life. A world in which poverty is endemic will always be prone to ecological and other catastrophes.

Meeting essential needs requires not only a new era of economic growth for nations in which the majority are poor, but an assurance that those poor get their fair share of the resources required to sustain that growth. Such equity would be aided by political systems that secure effective citizen participation in decision making and by greater democracy in international decision making.

(Brundtland Report, 1987: 8)

perspective of the problems facing the developing world – starvation, overpopulation, urbanisation, public health – and the environmentalist position which had begun to exercise the minds of so many in the developed world. In so doing, it attempted to bridge the divide between the green position that economic growth is harmful and the mainstream economic and political stance that growth is essential for the continuing harmony and prosperity of society. Brundtland's formulation of 'sustainable development' was acceptable across the political spectrum. From the developing country perspective, the report emphasised the essential needs of the world's poor, which the report stated should be accorded 'overriding priority'. From the green position, Brundtland adopted the idea of limits that would be imposed by the state of technology and social organisation on the ability of the environment to meet needs today and in the future.

Contained in the Brundtland definition is the idea of caring for future generations. Often described as environmental stewardship for future generations, this struck a new note in the environmental debate.

Given that a sustainable world is one where resources are used prudently, meaning that they will still be available for future generations, this can mean that a number of natural resources will be substituted by human-made products in order to conserve natural resources, although this too will necessitate the use of some other resources. Another way to restrict the use of resources of this kind – for example wood, coal, minerals – is to reduce the demand for them. For instance, consumers might be persuaded not to demand mahogany, with a consequent reduction in tree felling in the Brazilian rain forest. It is not only mineral resources that are threatened. It is also the animals and plants of the natural world that are endangered and need protection as they are hunted for meat, their fur or medicinal properties. Therefore, sustainability has to apply to humankind's relationship with the animal and plant world as well. It might be said that we should preserve species for the sake of our descendants, who should be able to live in a world where, for example, tigers and elephants still exist. Apart from this, species have their own right to exist, a right which is independent of the pleasure they afford to human beings or the meat they supply.

Sustainability also has a strong social justice component. If we wish, according to the definition, 'to meet the needs of the present', then those needs will include, at least in most people's understanding, the need to have adequate food, shelter and water. Many people in the world today do not have these necessities. The United Nations Food and Agriculture Organization estimates that there are 841 million people in the world – living in developing countries – who suffer from protein energy malnutrition, i.e. they do not receive sufficient protein calories. [But this is also a world where 600 million people are estimated to be overweight – 97 million of these are in the USA, where 55 per cent of the adult population is overweight, and the UK is not far behind with 51 per cent of its adult population being overweight (Brown in Brown and Flavin, 1999: 117]. There are more than fifty countries which are unable to provide safe water for domestic use, and 20 per cent of the world's population has only limited access to clean water because of pollution of the supply (Instituto del Tercer Mundo, 1997: 70; Carley and Spapens, 1998: 102). Adequate shelter is denied to 600 million people world-wide. Over 75 per cent of the world's population lives in developing countries, where urbanisation is proving to be a powerful magnet drawing people to the cities. Often, the only places they can find to live are illegal settlements on the outskirts, where they have to drink contaminated water and endure poor housing and health conditions (O'Meara in Brown and Flavin, 1999: 134). These basic resources for a civilised life are absent from many people's lives for numerous reasons: these include the working of an economic system which forces them to trade their crops on a world market for low prices or the fact that they live in a part of the world which is ill-favoured by nature, and they find it very hard to scratch a living because of drought and poor soil.

In the rich world, if we accept that we should restrain our use of natural resources for the sake of future generations, then we have to remember that, with the expected rise in world population from 6 billion to 9.4 billion by the year 2050, there will be many more people wanting those resources. If they were divided equally – which of course they will not be – then each person would receive less (L.R. Brown *et al.*, 1998). Sustainability involves taking a global perspective which includes consideration of the millions of people living in the poor world. This should mean the countries of the northern hemisphere taking fewer resources and living with fewer consumer goods. In fact, what has happened over the last quarter of a century has been the complete reverse with industrial societies using their increased wealth to enjoy even higher levels of consumption.

The rise of the consumer society

Since 1945, the majority of the population of the rich industrial nations have enjoyed a higher living standard than has ever been achieved before in world history. During the post-war years, labour-saving domestic appliances such as washing machines, fridges and vacuum cleaners found their way into working-class homes. With rising real incomes by the late 1950s, the 'affluent society' had emerged, and the Prime Minister Harold Macmillan could tell the British people in a famous phrase that 'you have never had it so good'. The affluent working class began to enjoy pleasures that were previously the exclusive preserve of the wealthy and the middle class. Cars and foreign holidays were now within the budget of many working people. In the 1950s and 1960s, the impact of a consumerist way of life on the natural environment was not discussed. But by the early 1970s, the mounting evidence of the damage that the industrial way of life was causing led a sizeable body of opinion to question the direction of advanced industrial societies.

The beginning of the contemporary concern with the environment dates from the early 1970s, when there was a real fear that the earth's stock of minerals and natural resources was going to be exhausted within a finite period coupled with the realisation of the damage which had already occurred to the environment. This was a recognition that economic growth had environmental consequences, although they might be experienced more by future generations than by contemporaries. The *Limits to Growth* report (Meadows *et al.*, 1972) was a landmark document warning industrial societies that time was running out for them as resources would only last for a finite period. The oil price rise by the Arab states in 1973 precipitated a crisis in the Western economic order which led to the first energy-saving measures – insulation, lower speed limits on the roads, reduction in the use of motor cars, some petrol rationing – during the period 1973–4. This coincided with the end of the long post-war boom in which employment levels had been high. This proved to be a temporary pause, however, as the growth of consumer societies and the era of cheap oil is still not at an end.

Over the past two decades, the growth of consumer societies has been unremitting, with newly industrialising countries aspiring to the range of goods and services which the people in the affluent First World enjoy. This consumption culture shows no signs of losing its fascination for the great majority of the population in First World countries. Shopping has become the principal leisure activity in the UK. The choice involved in consumption is at the heart of our society, and for many how we consume defines our identity just as much as the job that we do.

The emergence of a global communications network and a global market means consumer culture is now much more visible to the populations of the poor world, and rich world versions of the 'good life' appear to be increasingly influential. Consumerism has gone global. The growing popularity of long-distance air travel means that there are increasing encounters between rich and poor worlds, with the poor world chasing the dollars of the rich. Environmental consequences include the displacement of local people for the building of luxury hotels and golf courses, damage to the water table and the migration of people from the land to work in the tourist industries.

It is sobering to remember that one meaning of consume is 'to destroy'. Consumer societies are particularly damaging to the environment as their benefits depend upon the use of non-renewable energy: gas, electricity and oil. They generate vast quantities of waste by cultivating dissatisfaction among the population via the medium of advertising, which can only be assuaged by buying more goods. Twenty per cent of the world's population, mainly living in the West, consume 80 per cent of the world's resources (McLaren *et al.*, 1998: xiii). The vast quantities of goods to be found in the shops of the consumer societies have been manufactured from oil, coal, gas and other non-renewable resources. The production of consumer goods uses large amounts of energy; then when we have finally finished with these goods there is the problem of disposal. Households, commerce and industry in the UK create around 145 million tonnes of waste a year (Department of the Environment, Transport and the Regions, 1998a: 24).

Fred Hirsch's (1977) ground-breaking analysis in his book *The Social Limits to Growth* demonstrated that consumer goods are a positional good, i.e. they remain valued if they have a scarcity value; in this way they convey status or superiority. The classic example which he used was the motor car, pointing out that in its early days the motor car had a high positional advantage as there were so few other cars on the road – a scenario which many car advertisements portray today even though this is pure fantasy (Hirsch, 1977). Hirsch argued that the built-in restraints on the pursuit of self-interest which had been present in the nineteenth century had been eroded by consumer culture so that there was no longer a common set of values. Hirsch cited traffic congestion as an example of the positional economy. The satisfaction derived from an automobile depends on the traffic conditions in which it can be used, and these deteriorate as use becomes more widespread.

In modern consumer societies, the population is locked into a 'work and spend' cycle which is maintained by the cultivation of dissatisfaction by advertising agencies working on behalf of the consumer goods industries. Other satisfactions in life – family, friendship, hobbies – are sacrificed to the demands of paid work, which enables people to keep competing with others as consumers.

Economic growth

In the post-war period, the expansion of the social security system, the health service, social services and public housing was based upon the prospect of increasing economic growth. Economic growth provided the resources for social policy and removed the need to redistribute significant sums of money from the most affluent sections of the population in order to pay for the welfare state. This was convenient for government as increasing taxation to achieve this aim would have been electorally unpopular. The commitment to economic growth was to be found across the political spectrum from right to left and formed part of a post-war consensus which also embraced the welfare state and full employment. This was questioned by green parties, which began to emerge in the early 1970s and which maintained that the desire for growth, and the inexorable expansion of industrial societies, had itself become the problem. Greens questioned growth from a number of angles, pointing out that many of the goods produced were not beneficial for humankind, e.g. armaments or dangerous chemicals or nuclear fuel (Porritt, 1984: Ch. 4). Above all, they based their critique on the fact that there were finite resources on our planet and growth societies were creating environmental problems which were producing serious problems for all living things on the earth.

The increasing extraction of resources is still subject to physical constraints – the amount of natural minerals left. The population explosion means that the earth is home to over 6 billion people at the beginning of the twenty-first century, with an expected increase to 9 billion by 2050. Although it is clear that the authors of the *Limits to Growth* report (Meadows *et al.*, 1972) overestimated the rate at which stocks of resources would be extinguished, their case remains that resources are finite and demands are increasing. To cope with this requires a much more efficient and environmentally responsible use of resources.

The latest Club of Rome report, published in 1997, sets out innumerable ways in which this could be achieved, demonstrating that at least four times as much wealth could be extracted from the resources currently used. Even with the halving in resource use that they advocate, the problem of global warming will not be halted (Von Weizsacker *et al.*, 1997). There are other question marks to set against the commitment to economic growth from a green perspective. Policies which favour economic growth in developing countries can also be criticised for shifting control of natural resources, e.g. forests where native peoples work for a sustainable livelihood are taken over by companies who then employ the indigenous people as wage labourers (Korten, 1996: 43).

The concept of limits is a recurrent theme in green thinking, and it is directly contrary to some of the more optimistic variants of capitalist economic growth. The limits imposed by the need to stay within the carrying capacity of the planet mean that limits have to be observed in social and economic life. However, the conventional equation of gross national product – calculated from the market prices for which goods and services are sold – with the welfare of the population is belied by that fact that the populations of rich countries show no greater sense of subjective well-being than poor countries.

A green critique of this consumerist lifestyle has centred on the fact that consumer societies are *overconsuming* societies: they use much more of the world's resources than is equitable or sustainable. Two concepts illustrate this fact: environmental space and ecological footprint.

Environmental space

Environmental space embodies the concept of limits because it is a device which is used to reckon how an equitable distribution of resources could be achieved. There are three principles involved in the concept of environmental space: (1) it entails a commitment to living within the earth's resources; (2) it involves a global equality of access to the resources of the earth by all peoples; and (3) it maintains that production and consumption should enhance the quality of life within national and cultural diversity (for a full explanation, see Carley and Spapens, 1998: Ch. 4). When comparisons are made between the share of resources taken by the rich world and the poor world then it is clear that the former makes much greater demands upon nature and the planet's support systems. The increasing population of poor countries is a matter for concern as it threatens their fragile infrastructures, but it has to be set against the fact that the inhabitants of the rich world consume far more of the earth's resources. Environmental space refers to the share of the planet and its resources that humans can reasonably take; the share of the earth's resources that they can consume without depriving future generations. It is calculated by specifying certain key resources at the national level and examines what rate of resource use is sustainable. McLaren *et al.* (1998) have taken energy, land, forests, water, steel and aluminium, cement and chlorine and estimated the annual rate of use for each resource and then calculated how much of each resource the UK should be using by 2050 if it is only to take an equitable share in comparison with other countries.

The concept of environmental space is relevant to social policy because it is perfectly possible for poor countries to have good health and education services but have only a fraction of the lifestyle level enjoyed by the majority of people in the rich world – in other words, to take very little environmental space. In these countries, there is low sustainable resource use and low levels of non-renewable energy consumption but social indicators such as infant mortality, i.e. the number of deaths per thousand live births up to age 1 year, and life expectancy are far better than in other parts of the poor world (Carley and Spapens, 1998: 139–40). In the Indian state of Kerala, the gross domestic product per head is $300 per year, indicating that few industrial products are manufactured and hence it has low pollution levels, which means that the Keralese have a very low impact upon the environment. But on social indicators, Kerala compares favourably with the USA. It has a birth rate near the American average, a low infant mortality rate and male life expectancy of 70 years (Carley and Spapens, 1998: 140). Kerala is an example of a society where social policy has been used to obtain a reasonable quality of life, although Kerala is poor when measured in league tables of ownership of consumer durables.

Ecological footprint

The ecological footprint is the total land occupied by virtue of a person's consumption of produce from land, consumption of wood and use of land for absorbing waste and pollutants. These are then aggregated at city level or country level to show the impact on the land of that population size. For example, it has been estimated that the ecological footprint for London is 125 times its present area, or 21 million hectares, which is the entire productive land of the UK (Girardet, 1996a: 24). Environmental space is used to compare consumption of different kinds of resources. In contrast, ecological footprints are measured by converting all kinds of resource use to the equivalent in terms of land area.

The two concepts of environmental space and ecological footprint link the discussion of consumer societies to sustainability. They provide a scale against which the sustainable development policies of government can be measured. Social policy analysis has, since its inception, measured the extent of social inequality.

When we look at the distribution of environmental hazards and pollution, what we discover is that – generally – those who suffer most from these are those people who are disadvantaged in other ways.

Social and environmental inequality

It is the poorest who suffer disproportionately from environmental hazards. Air pollution kills 2.7 million people each year, 90 per cent of whom are in the developing world. Most of them will die in villages, not the cities, as a result of using fuel in their homes which contains toxic substances. Five million people die annually as a result of drinking dirty contaminated water; 3 million of these are children. In the UK, the poor tend to live in the areas with the worst traffic fumes. Most of the 32,000 Britons who die each year from cold are poor people living in badly insulated homes (Lean, 1998). These raw statistics are ample testimony to the fact that the poor suffer the most from environmental problems. Inequalities between the richest and the poorest in the world are worsening: consumption has increased sixfold in the last 20 years and has doubled in the last 10 years. People in Europe and North America now spend $37 billion a year on pet food, perfume and cosmetics. This sum of money would provide basic education, water and sanitation, basic health and nutrition for all those people who do not have it at present and there would still be $9 billion to spare (Elliot and Brittain 1998). These are examples of environmental injustice where the poor suffer more because they are poor.

Quality of life

Quality of life as a concept encompasses a huge agenda from the state of the environment to personal growth, health, economic rewards, satisfaction in life and psychological well-being. It has been used to challenge many of the basic presuppositions of consumer societies and has come to the fore as a reaction to the excesses of consumerism. Proponents of a more sustainable way of life argue that consumption should be put in its place – that it is not the whole purpose of life and that we should refrain from trying to meet non-material needs with material goods for this simply will not work. As Jacobs (1997) has pointed out, clean air, a quieter countryside and personal safety all contribute to our quality of life, but, as he remarks, the term quality of life needs extension to the level of society as well. Public provision of services is important for the quality of life. We can argue that there is an overall loss for society if the number of public libraries is halved. Although I myself may never normally use them, my children may wish to do so, and there may be times in the future when I would need to access information contained in the local library. Accordingly, the arguments for quality of life are made in terms of what people are going to gain from the process – they might have less to spend because of taxation to pay for these services but they will find that their overall quality of life has improved. In other words, our satisfaction with life is related to the safety of our streets, the upkeep of our parks and the appearance of our public spaces in addition to our salary or the make of our car. It is maintained that these all contribute to a person's overall sense of well-being. Quality of life has to be about the quality of our society as a whole and not only about the quality of an individual's life.

Improving the quality of life can be achieved by government providing a context in which it is easier for citizens to behave in environmentally responsible ways. Governments can discourage certain kinds of behaviour by taxing them, and through grants and subsidies can encourage other kinds of behaviour. There has been a long-standing green insistence that the way we live our lives affects the health of the planet – how we travel, how much we recycle, how we use energy – but most people need some encouragement to behave in environmentally responsible ways. Environmental taxation has an important role to play here in the transition to a more sustainable society, as does education, advertising and the other forms of persuasion open to government.

Part of the satisfaction that comes from owning consumer goods derives from the use of the product itself, and this is keenly appreciated when it is removed from us. The Bowler family, who in 1999 accepted the challenge laid down by Channel 4 of living in a turn-of-the-century London middle-class house without any of the twentieth-century 'mod cons' – no electric light, no shower, no electric kettle, no central heating and cooking everything on a range, quickly missed these labour-saving devices. For most of us, it is when the central heating breaks down or the car does not start that we are reminded of the considerable benefits of modern goods, but also how reliant on them we have become. Consumption is also a social process in which individuals participate, as Hirsch (1997) noted with his discussion of positional goods. Satisfaction can be derived from the status that consumer goods have within one's social circle. Designer clothing is highly rated by some people because it is meant to say something about you and to be noted by other people.

Quality of life has a subjective element. One person's view of what constitutes quality of life may be very different from another's. Realism also demands, however, that we acknowledge that in a consumer society our sense of subjective well-being and our needs are influenced – to a greater or lesser extent – by advertising and other techniques of persuasion.

Conclusion

Consumption cannot be overestimated as an important component of many people's life satisfaction. If the present pattern of consumption continues, there is little hope that we can avoid resource depletion and severe environmental problems in the next century, despite the fact that major advances are being made in the design of products which mean that they require far less energy input than was previously the case (Von Weizsacker *et al.*, 1997). The appeal of consumerism makes it unlikely that the majority of the population can be easily persuaded to reduce their levels of consumption.

The agenda for a sustainable social policy is daunting, for what is required is no less than a reduction in consumption by the majority of the population in the rich world. This is a reversal of the aspirations of most people in consumer societies. All the arguments about the environment and sustainability have to take account of the fact that we increasingly live in a global consumer society as more developing countries get sucked into the 'work and spend' way of life pioneered in the West.

As Bauman (1994) remarks:'consumption has seduced populations in the West and is now doing so in parts of the developing world'. There is much to suggest that the process of globalisation and privatisation of life-style will reinforce this ideology. An environmentally sensitive social policy, however, has the capacity to deliver a better quality of life. Social policy was regarded in the twentieth century as a means of producing greater social integration by reducing inequality, promoting citizenship and promoting social justice, and the sustainability agenda puts these ambitions in a new context. The challenge for social policy in the twenty-first century is to engage with sustainable development; the remainder of this book explores how this is being done.

Key points

- Social policy is an important component of sustainable development.
- Brundtland redefined the debate on the environment by emphasising the importance of meeting the needs of people in the present and in the future alongside environmental protection.
- Environmental space and ecological footprint are two useful methods of understanding the relationship between environmental limits and the distribution of resources.
- The concept of quality of life highlights the importance of public provision to individual well-being.

Guide to further reading

Carley, M. and Spapens, P. (1998) *Sharing the World: Sustainable Living and Global Equity in the 21st Century*, London: Earthscan. A clear exposition of the methods which can be used to achieve sustainable development.

Huby, M. (1998) *Social Policy and the Environment*, Buckingham: Open University Press. Demonstrates how consideration of the environment is fundamental to understanding of social policy.

Jacobs, M. (ed) (1998) *Greening the Millennium?*, Oxford: Blackwell. Contains an essay by Jacobs on the 'quality of life' and chapters on environmental politics and policy-making.

McLaren, D., Bullock, S. and Yousuf, N. (1998) *Tomorrow's World*, London: Earthscan. This is a Friends of the Earth book which argues that Britain has to make deep cuts in consumption so that developing countries can escape from poverty.

Social Policy and Administration (2001) 'Special issue: Environmental issues and social welfare', *Social Policy and Administration* 35, 5.

The Brundtland Report (The World Commission on Environment and Development) (1987) *Our Common Future*, Oxford: Oxford University Press. Essential reading as it sets out the sustainability agenda.

Chapter 2
Sustainable development
The policy response

Outline

This chapter outlines the ways in which the international community, the European Union and the UK government have responded to the agenda laid down by the Brundtland Report. It notes the different emphases of the Conservative and Labour governments and examines the sustainable development agenda of the Labour government, which combines social, economic and environmental objectives.

The Rio Summit

The Brundtland report paved the way for the United Nations Conference on Environment and Development (the Earth Summit) held in Rio de Janeiro in 1992. Representatives from 176 countries endorsed a programme of sustainable development designed to meet the challenge of world poverty and environmental crisis. In another part of Rio, at the same time, there was a huge gathering of people representing non-governmental organisations from around the world. The Earth Summit was a landmark in international environmental co-operation, although it did not fulfil many of the hopes invested in it by green activists.

The agreement reached at Rio committed each national government to the production of a sustainable development plan based on Agenda 21, the sustainability action strategy agreed at the summit. The Rio Summit also produced two other agreements: one on biodiversity, i.e. the variety and variability of living organisms, and one on climate change. It is the perspective of Agenda 21 which has done most to change the perception of sustainability among the policy community and which has obvious implications for social policy.

Agenda 21

All countries represented at the Rio Earth Summit signed the Agenda 21 declaration. This was in itself a major achievement, although it was open to various interpretations by national governments. The declaration is in four sections:

- social and economic dimensions which deal with the connections among poverty, consumption, debt, population and environmental problems;
- the conservation and management of resources for development – the means by which land, energy, the seas and waste can be used to further sustainable development;
- the ways in which major social groups can be brought into alliances around sustainable development;
- the implementation of Agenda 21.

It is important to note the limitations which correspond to the realities of power politics and the conflict between the rich and the poor worlds such that the USA was prepared to veto any action which would lead to any redistribution of economic power. Further, the fund which was established whereby rich countries would contribute to the costs incurred by poor countries in moving towards sustainable development has been notably short of donors (Connelly and Smith, 1999: 206–7). Although the follow-up Earth Summit held in New York in 1997 was disappointing in its outcomes, the fact remains that discussions of the environment are now automatically linked to questions of social justice, and it was the discourse of sustainability, endorsed at Rio, which achieved this.

The UK response to Rio

In the late 1980s, the Conservative government, led by Mrs Thatcher, responded to the growing alarm occasioned by mounting scientific evidence on global warming and climate change by preparing a White Paper, *This Common Inheritance* (Department of the Environment, 1990). This was largely a catalogue of existing environmental measures already being taken by the government. It was a disappointment to the green movement and did not reflect the thinking of one of the government's environmental advisers, Professor David Pearce, who had popularised the case for market-based solutions to environmental problems (Pearce, 1989). Pearce argued that each generation should pass onto the next a stock of assets no less than those it inherits. This stock would include environmental capital – clean air and water, ozone layer, coral reefs, etc. – and human-made capital – technology, the infrastructure of a country, etc. It would be possible to achieve trade-offs between the two, but only if the overall combined stock was not reduced. In pursuit of this analysis, Pearce advocated pricing environmental goods so that they would be used more prudently in the economy. It appears that industrialists who had the ear of the Conservative government used their influence to block these ideas. Although this particular approach suggested by Pearce was not adopted by the Conservative government, the use of economic concepts and methods is a defining feature of the ecological modernisation approach, which believes that it is possible to combine economic growth with environmental protection and which has become the consensual view of UK governments (see Chapter 4).

Rio gave a boost to environmental thinking within the Conservative government, which moved quickly to produce a national environmental plan in line with the Earth Summit declaration. *Sustainable Development: the UK Strategy* (Department of the Environment, 1994) did not represent an outline of new policy but instead brought together existing policy commitments into one document. The strategy established two new bodies: a Panel on Sustainable Development, composed of five experts who proffered advice to government, and a Roundtable on Sustainable Development, which was composed of representatives from voluntary organisations, business and interest groups in an attempt to build consensus on the best way forward on sustainable development. As noted by Connelly and Smith (1999: 265), the strategy broke with the market solutions of the Conservative government by endorsing demand management, although at other places in the document it contends that the government cannot impose restrictions on citizens; most significantly, there are no targets in the strategy. It is possible to argue that without the UK being committed to sustainable development some policy decisions may well not have occurred. In 1989, when Mrs Thatcher was Prime Minister, the Conservatives had launched the biggest road-building programme ever announced by a British government in order to cope with the projected increase in traffic. In 1996, the government made a U-turn on road building: many of the schemes were dropped, reflecting the government's new view that 'predict and provide' was not a sensible basis for transport policy and, furthermore, that the other less environmentally damaging modes of public transport – walking and cycling – would need to be actively promoted. Electoral considerations were possibly more important in coming to this decision, however, as the Conservatives were conscious that many of their traditional supporters in the shires were opposed to particular road-building schemes. Likewise, the government changed its mind on planning permission for out-of-town superstores – major generators of traffic – announcing in 1994 that no more planning permission would be given for these projects. However, this did not mean that no out-of-town stores were built after this date because there were many schemes still in the pipeline that had planning permission.

Undoubtedly, the most active and enthusiastic response to Rio in the UK came from those local authorities who adopted Agenda 21. UK local authorities have been among the pace-setters in the drive towards local sustainability. Local Agenda 21, with its all-inclusive approach to sustainability, gave local authorities a leadership role in their areas and enabled them to regain some of the legitimacy they had lost because of the relentless assault on them by the Thatcher government (see Chapter 3).

European Union environmental policy

As a supranational body with its own environmental policy, the European Union (EU) was a signatory to the Rio Summit declaration in 1992 and the Kyoto agreement in 1997. The EU, to which the UK has belonged since 1973, is a supranational organisation which currently encompasses 370 million people, but this will increase to over 500 million with the accession of countries in central and eastern Europe in the near future. Although there was no mention of the environment in the Treaty of Rome in 1957, which formed the European Economic Community, the precursor to the EU, environmental issues were put firmly on the agenda in the early 1970s. The Paris Summit of the European Community in 1972 declared that 'economic expansion is not an end in itself – it should result in an improvement in the quality of life as well as the standard of living' (Barnes and Barnes, 1999: 28). This led to a series of Environmental Action Programmes – of which the fifth, commencing in 1992, was a response to the Brundtland agenda and Rio. The Fifth Environmental Action Programme is the EU's sustainable development policy, entitled 'Towards Sustainability' (see Box 2.1). But it is important to recognise that it is not a policy which is compulsory for member states. Although criticised for being a weak version of sustainable development, it is a measure of how much beliefs have changed that the EU, established to facilitate trade relations between member states, can commit itself to a sustainable development strategy.

At the Council of Ministers there is qualified majority voting on some environmental issues, which means that member states cannot veto these measures. Those decisions which are adopted at the Council of Ministers do not have to go to the national parliaments for ratification.

The EU does not have enforcement powers, so it is reliant on member states ensuring that EU policy is being implemented. An inspectorate to ensure that member states comply with environmental legislation has been suggested but ruled out on the grounds of cost. Because the European Commission has had scarce independent information, the European Environment Agency was launched by the EU in 1993 with a mandate to orchestrate, cross-check and implement the use of information relevant to the protection of the environment. The biggest impact of the EU on environmental policy in the UK has been on the style of policy-making because the EU has insisted on certain standards being met, e.g. in air pollution this has led to greater centralisation and

Box 2.1 The Fifth EU Environmental Action Programme

Policy instruments
Legislation to set environmental standards
Economic instruments to encourage the production and use of environmentally friendly products and processes
Horizontal support measures (information, education, research)
Financial support measures (funds)

Five target areas
Industry
Energy sector
Transport
Agriculture
Tourism

Themes and targets
Climate change
Acidification and air quality
Urban environment
Coastal zones
Waste management
Management of water resources
Protection of Nature and bio-diversity
(European Commission, 1993)

closer monitoring of local authorities by central government (Garner, 2000).

Policy integration is now seen as key to achieving more real progress in improving the environment, as with the Fifth Environmental Action Programme. But there is little sign as yet that this has been forthcoming as policies in areas such as agriculture with the Common Agriculture Policy, transport with the Sustainable Mobility Policy – itself a contradiction in terms – and an energy policy can be said on many occasions to conflict with sustainable development. It would appear that member states are not prepared to countenance the degree of regulatory activity that policy integration for sustainable development would require.

New Labour: a 'green government'?

The Labour government elected in May 1997 provided a more extended version of sustainability than the Conservatives by linking it directly with the main programmes in other areas, including social policy. In so doing, this is in keeping with the emphasis on combating inequality to be found in Agenda 21. Labour announced itself as a green government; one of its first actions was to merge the Department of Transport with the Department of the Environment, thus creating a superministry – the Department of the Environment, Transport and the Regions (DETR), although they have since been decoupled. In his speech to the Earth Summit in New York shortly after coming to power, the Prime Minister Tony Blair declared: 'We must make the process of government green. Environmental considerations must be integrated into all our decisions, regardless of the sector' (Young 1998). The 'green ministers' – a minister in each department who has the responsibility for green issues, an idea inherited from the Conservatives – meet regularly and there is now a Parliamentary Audit Committee on the Environment to monitor progress. In a number of ways, Labour has pursued an environmental agenda with some vigour – at the Kyoto summit on global warming in 1997 and again at the Hague in 2000. The UK has been a major player in the move to reduce greenhouse gases and has pledged that the UK will reduce carbon dioxide emissions by 20 per cent of their 1990 levels by the year 2010.

It seems that Labour's big environmental test will be transport, an environmental issue where government can do so much with policy and expenditure but needs to persuade the public to change its travelling behaviour. The 1997 Labour manifesto stated: 'A sustainable environment requires above all an effective and integrated transport policy' (Labour Party, 1997). In its White Paper on Transport published in the summer of 1998, Labour spelt out its commitment to an integrated transport system with restrictions on car use envisaged and clear priority given to walking, cycling and public transport (Department of the Environment, Transport and the Regions, 1998b). Coming to power with a strong belief in the contribution of public transport but without an electoral mandate to renationalise the railway system, Labour has significantly boosted the powers of the rail regulator, and in its 10-year plan for transport announced in 2000 (Department of the Environment, Transport and the Regions, 2000) it has greatly increased expenditure on public transport. But New Labour was elected because it correctly understood the psychology of the electorate and some of the more radical measures to reduce car use were reportedly dropped from the document because they would be seen as 'anti-car' and therefore unpopular with large sections of the voting public. The government has backed away from the challenge of introducing a national road-pricing scheme and other measures designed to cut car dependence, instead giving these powers to local authorities. It appears that few local authorities will wish to use these powers for fear of discouraging shoppers and inward investment. Without these measures, car use and car ownership will continue to grow, exacerbating global warming and pollution levels. It is difficult to see how the government can deliver on its promised 20 per cent cut in carbon dioxide emissions without reducing the volume of traffic on the roads with measures of this kind.

Quality of life

The publication of *A Better Quality of Life: A strategy for sustainable development for the UK* (Department of the Environment, Transport and the Regions, 1999a) pursued the theme that social and environmental policy are inter-related. The government has defined sustainable development as: 'a better quality of life for everyone, now and for generations to come'. The mixing of social and environmental policy is seen in the objectives it declares: 'social progress which recognises the needs of everyone', 'effective protection of the environment', 'prudent use of natural resources' and the 'maintenance of high and stable levels of economic growth and employment' (Department of the

Environment, Transport and the Regions, 1999a). The document outlines the ways in which the government is committed to ensuring that sustainable development is built into its main policies and programmes. Across all these diverse areas the government has announced indicators by which its progress can be judged (see Box 2.2).

The strategy embodies a New Labour analysis of the way the world is heading as it is committed to high levels of economic growth and a highly skilled workforce, recognising that much industrial production is now being carried out in the poor world. The document points to the greater productivity of workers in the USA and France and Germany and stresses the need for much better educational attainment in a knowledge economy. We will explore these themes in Chapter 9.

The Labour government's sustainable development policy is not only to be found in the pages of its strategy. The Regional Development Agencies that the government has established have a brief to produce regional sustainability plans. Although *A Better Quality of Life* (Department of the Environment, Transport and the Regions, 1999a) has a chapter entitled 'A sustainable economy', it makes no mention of environmental taxation – taxing industries

---

Box 2.2 Government's headline indicators

Total output of the economy (GDP)
Investment in public, business and private assets
Proportion of people of working age who are in work
Qualifications at age 19 years
Expected years of healthy life
Homes judged unfit to live in
Level of crime
Emissions of greenhouse gases
Days when air pollution is moderate or high
Road traffic
Rivers of good or fair quality
Populations of wild birds
New homes built on previously developed land
Waste arisings and management

(DETR, 1999a)

which pollute and moving away from taxation on jobs, such as the national insurance contributions. However, soon after coming to power, the government announced its intention to introduce environmental taxation. This resulted in the 1999 budget announcement that increases in fuel duties beyond inflation would be 'ring-fenced' for transport spending. In addition, a tax on industrial use of energy was introduced, which means that all coal, gas and electricity bills will have a sum added for the climate change levy. The aim is not to raise money but rather to get industry to reduce its use of energy. National insurance contributions from employers are being reduced to off-set the cost to them.

The sustainable development agenda

Although the Rio Summit was billed as an opportunity for the international community to respond appropriately to the evidence on climate change, the destruction of the ozone layer and species extinction, progress has been slow and disappointing. The vision of sustainable development has, however, provided a new context for government policy-making. The Conservative government had a distaste for planning, which meant that it was lukewarm in its support for sustainable development although some individual ministers were extremely committed. The Labour government, in contrast, is much more committed to the sustainable development agenda – particularly to social policy, which features heavily in its strategy document. Yet the omissions should be noted: there is no discussion of sustainable consumption, no mention of environ-mental space or the ecological footprint. From its performance since 1997, it would appear that the Labour government is not instinctively green. New Labour would appear to mistrust the environmental agenda because it associates it with utopian green thinking (Jacobs, 1999). The government seems to believe that it would be courting electoral unpopularity if it were to take radical measures to protect the environment such as those mentioned above, which would have made motoring more expensive. Because the government monitors public opinion closely, it is aware that although it uses the term sustainable development in relevant documents the public is largely ignorant as to what it means. The challenge remains for this government – indeed, the democratic system – to lead public opinion towards acceptance of restraints on some forms of environmentally damaging behaviour because the environmental crisis demands it. In the next chapter, we outline the response of local authorities to sustainable development.

Key points

- The Rio Summit committed each nation to a sustainable development strategy.
- The Conservatives' sustainable development strategy did not result in major policy initiatives.
- The European Union's Fifth Environmental Action Programme was not binding on member states and lacked targets.
- Labour has introduced sustainability indicators and targets for sustainable development.

Guide to further reading

Books on the politics of sustainable development date quickly because of the changing nature of institutions and policy-making.

The best way to keep up to date on government policy-making in this area is regularly to access the World-Wide Web – Department of the Environment, Food and Rural affairs (www.defra.gov.uk); Commission for Sustainable Development (which replaced the Panel and Round Tables) (www.sd-commission.gov.uk). Also check the government's sustainable development site (www.sustainable-development.gov.uk).

For a critical response to sustainable development policy, monitor the Friends of the Earth web site (www.foe.org).

Chapter 3
Local Agenda 21

Outline

This chapter introduces Local Agenda 21 (LA 21), which is the local strategy for sustainable development. Local authorities who have endorsed LA 21 have been working with other parts of the public sector together with residents and business and voluntary organisations to create a 'shared vision' of what is required for sustainability. This has produced a great many assessments both of social need and of the priorities for the local environment and sustainability. A major theme has been the participation of groups that traditionally have not been included in the political process. LA 21 provides interesting examples of a marriage between environmental and social policy.

Introduction

The Agenda 21 document agreed at the Rio Earth Summit in 1992 declared that humankind should share wealth and opportunities more fully between the northern and southern hemispheres, between countries, and between different social groups within each country, with special emphasis on the needs and rights of the poor and disadvantaged. It stated that this kind of change will only be realised by the process of democracy and participation: 'We will not achieve sustainable development by accident but must consciously plan and work for it, at all levels from international to local; all people, including poor and disadvantaged groups, must have a say in decisions about environment and development; all social groups and interests, including business, education, and voluntary and community groups as well as governments at all levels, will need to work in partnership' (United Nations, 1992). Central to Agenda 21 is the belief that sustainable development can only be achieved if deprived communities in the rich world together with the great majority of people living in low-income countries are given social and economic assistance. The LA 21 document recognises that unless this is done then there will be little support for sustainability from these communities or countries. It stated that environment policy should be integrated into decision-making at all levels and environmental improvement must be linked to improving the economic and social status of deprived communities. Agenda 21 stipulated that over half the required policy steps should be implemented in the locality, reflecting the view held by greens that planetary problems require local as well as national and international action.

Local environmental policy

In the UK, Local Agenda 21 built on the existing environmental policy and planning of local authorities. Environmental policy can be traced right back to the creation of local authorities in the mid-1830s, when they were established in order to deal with the social and environmental problems created by the industrial revolution and urbanisation. The emphasis in LA 21 on the merging of social and environmental policy is one that local authorities do not find unusual as they have had this range of responsibilities throughout their history. Public health was the main priority among the early responsibilities of local authorities, with housing, social welfare and education becoming local government services later in the nineteenth century.

In the 1980s, some local authorities had been at the forefront of greening and environmental initiatives. By 1991, the year before LA 21 was announced, 70 per cent of local authorities had adopted an environmental plan. It might be said that in this way they were claiming a leadership role in relation to environmental policy in their area. Most of these plans covered such topics as energy, pollution, recycling and waste, nature conservation, planning and transport. A minority did make reference as well to health, purchasing policy, environmental education and agriculture. There were environmental charters setting out broad principles concerning the environment and action plans committing the local authority to deadlines in relation to certain environmental objectives. It was common for a council to produce an internal policy impact statement which examined the ways in which the local authority's policies affected the local environment (Ward, 1993). But it took LA 21 and the concept of sustainability to begin the integration of social policy into the local environmental agenda.

The diversity in size and character of local authorities – ranging from large urban to small rural – makes it unsurprising that some have become more involved in sustainable development than others. Under the Conservative governments of John Major (1990–7), it was a policy area where the local authorities could take the initiative as this was not forthcoming from Whitehall. Some local authorities had moved into environmental policy – as distinct from their environmental services such as environmental health and housing – in the 1980s, before LA 21 emerged, because it enlarged their sphere of influence. During the Major years, despite the clear social policy emphasis in LA 21, there was much less impact on social services, on anti-poverty strategies, on housing, on tourism and on economic development.

Local authorities and Local Agenda 21

It has been claimed that LA 21 was 'the most significant shot in the arm for UK local government for many years' because it gave local authorities an important issue upon which they could take the lead, thus bolstering their legitimacy as the authentic voice of the local area and community (Christie, 1996). It came after a period during which local government was subject to substantial reorganisation and the way in which services were provided was changed considerably. The Conservative governments led by Mrs Thatcher between 1979 and 1990 altered the financial relationship between Whitehall and the local authorities. The result of this being that most of the revenue raised by local authorities is now determined by central government, both as to how much money can be raised and upon which services it will be spent. The Thatcher governments aimed to transform the role of local authorities from providers to enablers, meaning that they should not provide the services but rather enable the private sector, or the voluntary sector, to provide the services. The local authority role was to inspect and monitor the quality of services provided.

Integrating sustainability issues into the policy-making work of the local authority was an opportunity under the Conservative governments of John Major to widen the remit of local authorities and make connections between local authority departments, such as transport, and agencies, such as the health authority, which had in some areas literally never previously spoken to each other. There were increasing calls for linkages to be made between different policy areas and to recognise the interconnectedness of social policy as it impinged upon the lives of ordinary citizens. The New Labour government elected in 1997 made plain its intention to link policy areas and to produce 'joined up government'. Since 1997, welfare state services have been encouraged to co-operate on joint projects. In this context, 'joined up government' means local agencies co-operating on problems with which all of them are concerned in some way or another and entails them working closely with other agencies and involving them in their plans. This is being done through a variety of area-based strategies such as health action zones (see Chapter 5), education action zones and the new deal for communities, which are all targeted on areas with a high degree of social deprivation.

Within health improvement programmes, environmental topics such as air quality and transport are recognised as being relevant to the health chances of individuals and as being, furthermore, an important component of health inequality.

Local Agenda 21 is a very ambitious agenda for local government as it has so many wide-ranging aims and objectives, many of which go right beyond the traditional sphere of local government work. One of the most ambitious is the goal of involving all sectors of the community in creating a local sustainable society. As we saw in the previous chapter, the architects of Agenda 21 were only too well aware of the fact that certain groups tended not to be involved in traditional local government consultation so they designated them stakeholder groups – with whom local authorities were expected to consciously make links and alliances. Participation was crucial, for it has to be borne in mind that the vision behind LA 21 was for the local area to achieve sustainable development; it was always meant to be more than another local authority programme.

The Local Agenda 21 process

The key areas are outlined in Box 3.1.

Integrating sustainability issues

The authors of LA 21 were aware that there was a great danger that it would be confined to an environmental ghetto, therefore it was important to ensure that there was a commitment to LA 21 right throughout the local authority. Many local authorities had environmental plans, but the process of consultation which was entailed in LA 21 meant that these were extended and refined through debate, deliberation and consultation. Some local authorities have produced State of the Environment reports, which look at the environmental problems of their area as a whole and not just at the services for which the local authority is responsible. An important part of the LA 21 process is the gathering of data on

---

Box 3.1 **The Local Agenda 21 Process**

Managing and improving the local authority's sustainability performance
Integrating sustainability issues into the local authority's policies and activities
Awareness raising and education
Consulting and involving the wider community and the general public
Working in partnership with others – central Government agencies, business, community groups and the general public
Measuring, monitoring and reporting

(Bateman, 1995)

environmental indicators and the setting of environmental targets. These are now called sustainability indicators, and we will return to them later in the chapter. Finally, LA 21 as part of the local authority enterprise had to be made part of its processes, and therefore it had to have targets and a mechanism established which would review them: 'To be effective, Agenda 21 needs to be part of a corporate strategy which is able to carry the underlying principles of environmental policy into the policy process across the authority' (Fodor *et al.*, 1995: 23). This would appear to be crucial, for the credibility of Agenda 21 depends upon local authorities setting a good example not only with their environmental policy but also with their practice. Clearly, the local authority which puts environmental policies into force in its own management and organisation will be more persuasive when it attempts to promote LA 21 with employers, voluntary organisations and the general public.

Awareness raising and education

Local authorities who are signed up to LA 21 need to canvass as wide a range of views as possible; it is for this reason that relying on the traditional (nineteenth century) model of representative democracy where the councillor speaks on behalf of the people is no longer feasible. Participation in local government elections is low, with a turnout of 25 per cent of the electorate not being uncommon. Because of this electoral apathy, the local authorities' claim to represent local people is weakened. Naturally, they have become keen to increase the participation of the public in local government. It is difficult for many people to participate, and this may not solely be the result of apathy: lack of time, lack of confidence and ignorance of the political process are contributory factors. Local Agenda 21 has used many different means to consult the local electorate: visioning, focus groups, community consultations and 'planning for real' are some of them. Visioning is a process where people from a local area are brought together in order to ascertain their hopes and fears for the future, in their district and nationally and internationally. 'Planning for real' involves making a three-dimensional model of the area, say 5 metres by

2.5 metres, which is then exhibited at various locations: community centres, schools and anywhere else that local people gather. Council officials attend these events and discuss the proposals with members of the public. They represent a significant variation on the representative model of democracy, in which it was one councillor who had the task of representing an area. But these, like voting, rely on people making an effort to participate, and this will only ever be a minority. For this reason, many local authorities make quite extensive use of market research firms in order to gauge what the majority think. There are two versions of democracy involved in this process: representative democracy, via the councillor elected for each ward, and participatory democracy, where individuals and groups get involved themselves in the decision-making process (Selman, 1996).

Community participation

Participation is key to Local Agenda 21 as sustainable policies are not going to work successfully unless they have widespread support. A shared understanding of what sustainability entails has had to be created. Local authorities have spent a lot of effort in consultation exercises to work out what sustainability would mean in their area. These endeavours are difficult, for the existing inequalities of knowledge, skills and confidence come to the fore. Articulate middle-class people find it easiest to participate and the recognition of this fact has led to a stress on 'capacity building', a term used in Agenda 21. This refers to helping people to achieve the skills and confidence necessary to participate, but it could equally be about the necessity of local authority professionals to hold back and allow local people to express their views on what is needed. If they are to consult effectively, then they may require new skills and approaches. Capacity building can also mean developing social capital, which is the web of social relationships linking citizens in the community. There are many ways of measuring social capital – membership of voluntary organisations in the broadest sense would be a guide so that bowls clubs, choral societies and chess clubs would be included just as much as church membership or the Girl Guides. These organisations and the myriad of clubs and societies have been identified as an index of how strong social relationships are within an area. Face-to-face relationships are key to social capital. One could argue that the number and extent of these voluntary organisations is an index of the strength of a community.

Partnership

LA 21 has brought together voluntary organisations in a local authority area in order to enlist them in the LA 21 process while recognising that they are but one group of stakeholders, i.e. the organisations affected by LA 21 or that wish to influence the programme. There are many other stakeholders who need to be brought into the process, and Table 3.1 gives an indication of how broad the range can be.

As part of the government's modernisation plans for public services, the White Paper *Modern Local Government* (Department of the Environment, Transport and the Regions, 1998d) proposed:

- ensuring policy-making is more joined up and strategic;
- making sure that public sector users are the focus by matching services more closely to people's lives;
- delivering public services that are of high quality and efficient.

Many local authorities have incorporated LA 21 into the new auditing procedures so that there is a LA 21 audit conducted as part of this process to monitor where the authority has reached. Some local authorities have incorporated LA 21 monitoring into their 'Best Value' programme, which replaced 'Compulsory Competitive Tendering' as a way of improving public sector purchasing and service provision.

Social deprivation

Sustainability involves a commitment to working towards the alleviation of poverty. LA 21 has been designed to ensure that linkages are made between environmental policy and the needs of people living in poor areas. For some time, environmentalists have

Table 3.1 Stakeholder groups

Community	Business	Public authorities and utilities	Cross-sectoral
Resident associations	Chambers of commerce	Local authorities	Schools, colleges, universities
Community groups	Chambers of trade	Parish councils	Community health councils
Councils for voluntary service	Industry organisations	Health authorities	Political parties
Urban wildlife and	Individual industries	Energy utilities	Trade unions
environment groups		Training and enterprise	Housing associations
Religious groups		councils	Campaigning organisations
Arts and recreation		Transport providers	Transport consultative
Minority ethnic groups			committees
Women's groups			

Source: adapted from Freeman *et al.* (1996).

faced the charge that it is only the affluent and the middle class who care about environmental issues as the rest of the population are too busy earning their living or looking for work. Serious attempts have been made with LA 21 to involve poor communities, which has meant LA 21 being translated into a language that everyone could understand. When council officials asked people in these deprived communities what was wrong with their environment, they told them about the broken lifts, the graffiti on the walls, the vandalised playground, the fear of going out at night because of mugging, the heavy traffic and the lack of safe places for children to play. These were the kinds of concerns that local residents had about their 'environment', by which of course they meant the built environment in which they lived. Clearly, many people in inner-city areas and outer estates feel that they have a poor quality of life. In other words, the real issues that annoy people about their local environment in inner-city areas and outer estates are related to the low wages, high unemployment and poverty that are to be found there. Local Agenda 21 is about tackling this essentially social policy agenda. To quote the Agenda 21 document on the objectives listed under 'Combating poverty', 'To develop for all poverty-stricken areas integrated strategies and programmes of sound and sustainable management of the environment, resource mobilization, poverty eradication and alleviation, employment and income generation' (United Nations, 1992: Ch. 3). Some of the sustainability indicators used by local authorities try to capture this. For example, Lancashire County Council has developed a set of thirty-nine sustainability indicators, and these include basic services within walking distance, distance travelled to work, homelessness, prosperity and deprivation, lead in drinking water, house prices, poverty and children in poverty (Lancashire County Council, 1997).

The people who live in poor areas will often have had their environment determined for them, not only in the sense that the houses and flats were usually built without considering the wishes of the residents but, to take one example, it is also often these areas that are chosen to take the new roads which will ease traffic congestion in other parts of the city. Despite its ambitions on the ground in inner-city areas, Local Agenda 21 is but one programme and is part of a wide spectrum of initiatives which includes crime prevention, anti-poverty strategies and in some areas the education and health action zones introduced by central government.

Sustainability indicators

How do we measure progress towards a sustainable society? How will we know when we have actually arrived at the promised land of sustainability? Will we all be able to agree that this is sustainability? These are difficult questions which have been the subject of considerable discussion since the sustainability debate went live with the publication of the Brundtland Report in 1987. Agenda 21 envisaged that sustainability indicators would represent a way by which individuals, communities, groups and institutions could make better choices about their futures.

A sustainability indicator is a measure which, taken with other measures, should show the progress or otherwise on the way to a sustainable society. These can be existing statistics or they can be statistics which are specially created for the task. For example, in measuring the progress towards a sustainable transport system, a range of existing statistics would be of assistance and these would include the amount of tiny particulates in the air (PM 10s), the serious injury rates on the roads, the number of fatalities, the number of vehicles using the roads, the number of people who use public transport and the number of people who cycle and who walk; along with all these figures, which are available from local and national sources, local people might also want to construct some statistics of their own. These might include the number of children who walk to school and the number of people who use the town's cycleways. Proponents of sustainability indicators believe that it is important for the community to create, where possible, its own indicators as then the exercise becomes more meaningful (MacGillivray,, 1998).

Lawrence (1998) distinguishes three kinds of indicator:

- *Distinct indicator.* This is a numerical representation of a condition or problem. The unemployment rate is a distinct indicator. The infant mortality rate is another, as is the percentage of unfit dwellings.

- *Comparative indicator.* This is a good way of giving more meaning to distinct indicators. They can be compared with distinct indicators elsewhere. For example, infant mortality rates or the percentage of unfit housing can be compared between cities. This can sometimes lead to action, for no one – certainly not a politician – wants to be at the bottom of a league table.

- *Directional indicators.* This usually means that a benchmark statistic is decided upon, and then the progress towards this is measured. For example, it might be decided that there should be classes of only twenty pupils in each primary school in the country, and progress towards this could be measured in each school and local education authority area.

There is much in the literature on sustainability indicators which says that they have to be owned by the community, meaning that the community decides what it values and holds individuals accountable. Proponents argue that sustainability indicators should encourage greater democracy by enabling people to measure what they think is important (Bell and Morse, 1999: 66).

In local authority areas all over the country, there have been sustainability indicator exercises. These, like the LA 21 process itself, have tried to involve as many people and groups as possible, with community and campaigning organisations being invited to play a part in the process and to suggest ideas for the indicators themselves. The Sustainability Indicators Research Project of the Local Government Management Board proposed 101 draft indicators grouped around the following thirteen themes:

- efficient use of resources;
- limiting pollution;
- diversity of nature to be valued;
- local needs to be met locally;
- everyone to have access to food, water, shelter and fuel;
- opportunities for work;
- good health;
- access to facilities and services;
- freedom from fear of crime and persecution;

- access to skills, knowledge and information;
- involvement in decision-making;
- opportunities for culture available to all;
- places and spaces combining meaning and beauty with utility.

Sustainability indicators are meant to represent the way in which individuals and groups can make better choices about their futures, with the expectation that the indicators would lead to a change in behaviour. There is as yet little evidence of this. Lawrence (in Dodds, 1997: 183) believes that this is because the wider community has not been involved in deciding which statistics to collect. 'In large part it is because few of us are willing to change our behaviour which is based upon someone else's determination of meaning' (Lawrence in Dodds, 1997: 183). This may well be the case for some people, but there are complex reasons as to why we persist in behaviour which is damaging to the environment. There will always be a small number of people who will change their behaviour as a result of sustainability indicators or environmental reports. The optimism of the Agenda 21 authors when they assumed that there will be majority support for sustainable development was possibly misplaced.

Conclusion

A Friends of the Earth survey of councillors, officials and others involved in LA 21 found that they believed that even in those authorities which had the appropriate planning machinery there were still innumerable barriers to seeing the implementation of LA 21 plans. It was claimed that there was a lack of political will in local authorities, and there was some scepticism as to how far central government would push sustainability against the perceived opposition of some parts of the electorate. There were also fears that electoral considerations would mean that implementation of LA 21 was delayed. Many councillors had little understanding of what sustainability entailed. Among other barriers was the view that many people felt that on occasions the divide would be between jobs and the environment (Friends of the Earth, 1998).

Although the obstacles to an effective implementation of LA

21 are real enough, they should not detract from the fact that Agenda 21 is a major document which, by its very nature, will take years to implement. It gives concrete shape to the platform of the Brundtland Report, namely that environmental and socioeconomic issues had to be interlinked and that there would be no real movement on environmental issues unless they were integrated with economic and social policy. It is an index of how great is the magnitude of the task facing humankind in the transition to a sustainable society.

Local Agenda 21 on its own cannot achieve that fusion of social, economic and environmental policy which is needed to make sustainability much more of a reality in the UK. It does, however, provide a remarkably good tool by which local authorities can initiate a debate in their area about sustainability. The traditional environmental areas such as waste management, countryside and biodiversity and land-use planning have been most affected by the Local Agenda 21 programme. Nonetheless, it has definitely moved social policy onto the sustainability agenda. Community participation has been a central feature of LA 21 since its inception on the premise that sustainability policy had to show the relevance of environmental concerns to other areas of social and economic policy. LA 21 has to be popularised, otherwise, as several commentators have noted, there will not be the support for environmental and social policies, including the reduction in consumption patterns, which will be required in the twenty-first century. There is a danger that participation can reinforce the existing patterns of social inequality, with the articulate middle class having the wherewithal and skills to take part while other sections of the population do not have a voice at the meetings and workshops because they are absent. The participation of local residents in deprived areas is critical if the quality of life there is to be improved. There are many examples where communities have not been consulted and environmental schemes have been imposed from above and then vandalised (Taylor, 1998: 14). How to integrate the new ways of obtaining local views and local participation with the electoral process will be a serious challenge for local government.

O'Riordan and Voisey (1998: 232) outline five key elements in Local Agenda 21:

- multi-sectoral involvement in the preparation of long term sustainable development plans;
- consultation with local people creates a 'shared vision' and a mechanism for the identification of problems;
- participatory assessment of local social and economic conditions and needs;
- participatory target setting;
- monitoring and reporting procedures.

With its stress on democratic participation, Local Agenda 21 is working against the grain of a society where there is mounting evidence of apathy and alienation from political systems (O'Riordan and Voisey, 1998). The small number of people who know what the term sustainability means is some index of how great an awareness there is in the wider society.

No one could accuse the authors of Agenda 21 of a lack of ambition. Agenda 21 proposes changes in the way we live our lives – including how we spend our leisure time and how we travel – to accommodate the demands of sustainability. It is not easy to achieve behavioural change on this scale. It remains an open question whether it will be possible to achieve this in a consumer society where the dominant messages reinforce an unsustainable way of life based upon profligate energy use. Macnaghten and Urry (1998) claim that their research on attitudes to environmental problems 'suggests that people do express mounting concern over the trajectory of their society, including a pronounced and widespread pessimism over the future'. However, they note that among their respondents 'There was a notable absence in all the discussions of the view that markets, technological advances or political foresight would ameliorate current or future environmental problems. By contrast, the dominant claim was the inevitability of a more polluted and dangerous environment' (Macnaghten and Urry, 1998: 230).

This is in contrast to the early years of environmental awareness in the 1970s, when there was much faith in the ability of technology and government to solve environmental problems. Yet, despite this big shift in attitude towards government's role and the loss of belief in technological solutions to environmental problems, there is little evidence of a shift in personal behaviour. Macnaghten and Urry do not report that there has been a corresponding acceptance that because governments cannot be expected to deal effectively with these problems then individuals have to do this themselves. In general, they found that people do not feel that they can do much personally. Furthermore, the state is seen as part of the problem and many people do not trust official statistics, so this again makes a local authority-led initiative such as LA 21 more difficult. If these findings are true for a larger section of the population, then they are a measure of the distance that LA 21 has to cover.

None of this is to deny that LA 21 represents an important step forward in the transition to sustainability by its marriage of social and environmental concerns and by its emphasis on partnership and participation. Indeed, the new roles which many LA 21 local authorities have taken in partnership with deprived communities in supporting local employment trading systems, credit unions and a variety of environmental improvement organisations represents a significant boost to the 'social economy', as we shall see in Chapter 7 (Young, 1997).

Key points

- Many local authorities in the UK have introduced imaginative and effective ways to make sustainability part of the local political life.
- The use of sustainability indicators represents a valuable means of encouraging the debate on the future of local areas.
- Many of the key topics identified as important by local people in LA 21 are social policy issues.

Guide to further reading

Carley, M. and Christie, I. (2000) *Managing Sustainable Development*, London: Earthscan. An authoritative account of sustainable development with numerous case studies.

Dodds, F. (ed.) (1997) *The Way Forward: Beyond Agenda 21*, London: Earthscan. A collection of essays that examine the main themes of Local Agenda 21.

Dodds, F. (ed.) (2000) *Earth Summit 2002: A New Deal*, London: Earthscan. Written in preparation for the Johannesburg Earth Summit 2002 ('Rio plus 10'), which will review progress on Agenda 21 and set new targets for a global sustainable development strategy.

Selman, P. (1996) *Local Sustainability*, London: Paul Chapman. A discussion of the ways in which citizens, organisations and business can respond to the challenge of Local Agenda 21.

Warburton. D. (ed.) (1998) *Community and Sustainable Development*, London: Earthscan. Shows how participation can extend democracy, citizenship and accountability.

Web sites

The Department of Transport, Local Government and the Regions (DLTR) has extensive material on Local Agenda 21 including the Community Strategy, which local authorities have to prepare under the Local Government Act 2000 as part of their responsibility for measures that promote 'environmental well-being' (www.dltr.gov.uk).

Improvement and Development Agency (I&DEA) is worth visiting and has a variety of LA 21 links (www.la21-uk.org.uk).

There is a government web site devoted to sustainability indicators (www.sustainable-development.gov.uk/indicators/index.htm).

For papers and links on indcators and associated topics see the New Economics Foundation site (www.neweconomics.org).

Chapter 4
Green ideas

Outline

Green ideas come from a range of different origins and many have been around since the nineteenth century. This chapter provides a brief guide to green ideas from the dark greens who believe that industrialisation was a mistake right through to the ecological modernisers who think that capitalism can go green.

Introduction

Ideologies are sets of principles or ideas which can help us to organise our world. Often, they are regarded as common sense; they can simplify things and, at times, reduce the need to think. This can be harmful: the appalling consequences of a blind commitment to ideology are the twentieth century's concentration camps. Green thinking has until recently been about the future, creating a world which is much more in harmony with nature. To simplify a complicated issue, we can say that there are two possible responses to the ecological crisis facing humankind. One is denial: carry on consuming, carry on having fun and forget about our responsibility for the future. Or, we can imagine a green future where nature would not be subjected to a daily assault from humankind's cars, planes and way of life and where animals would not be slaves to the dinner plate mentality of human beings. There is much green thinking which takes this position, but in a variety of ways and from a number of different starting points. In some ways, green thought is the obvious successor to the socialism and communism of the twentieth century. Inspired by these ideologies,

millions of people worked to realise a society where there would
be a fair distribution of goods and services, and often this would
just mean that there would be simply enough to eat. Frequently,
they would be dismissed as idealists, and the most common
response was that these ideas were impractical and went against
human nature. In this chapter, we will examine a range of
ideologies, most of which would have this charge levelled against
them as well as ideologies which are more pragmatic. The latter
have been mixed with contemporary political ideas on the Right
and the Left so that they represent subsets of liberalism, socialism
or conservatism. This chapter examines the roots of green thinking
and then outlines the forms that green thought has taken in the
contemporary world.

No end to ideology

With the collapse of communist governments across Eastern Europe
and in the Soviet Union in 1989, there was a corresponding claim
in the West that finally we had seen an end to ideology. The
headlines were: 'Cold war over – the West has won'. The battle
between capitalism and communism was over – capitalism had
triumphed. There was, of course, a great deal of truth in this as the
market as a way of organising human affairs was an extremely
powerful idea, which coupled with consumerism appealed to the
people of Eastern Europe and the former Soviet Union. Globally,
the market system was advancing, spreading its tentacles to new,
emerging, industrialising countries, and in the Far Eastern
economies there were examples of very high growth rates. But in
reality, there was no end to ideology, for the critiques of capitalism
still existed although socialism and communism had lost much of
their appeal. Besides which, it was difficult to maintain that there
was an end to ideology when Islam, for example, had such a hold
over countries and people throughout the world.

The ideology of consumer capitalism has been an extremely
powerful advertisement for the market system and for capitalism.
Its ability to blend freedom, sexuality and power into consumer
products has been so seductive that in the UK today none of the
major political parties dares to challenge the consumer society –

their focus groups would tell them that it would be electoral suicide. As religious belief has dwindled in advanced industrial societies, the yearning, hopes and aspirations which previously were channelled into religion and its disciplines of prayer, charity and religious observance are now expressed within consumerism. As Bocock (1993: 50) has written, consumerism is 'the active ideology that the meaning of life is to be found in buying things and pre-packaged experiences'. Just as Christianity had the soul, the key to the belief system of the new religion is the self. This self is pandered to by consumer products that promise the illusion of happiness. The ideology of consumerism is so powerful that it is subscribed to by all sorts and conditions of people from across the political spectrum. We should not forget, however, that the climate in which the ideas in this chapter are discussed is one where the consumer society is seen as natural and desirable (see Miles, 1998). In previous centuries, the rich have had a monopoly of consumption, but over the last four decades mass consumer societies have emerged which have had the effect of deepening the environmental crisis and at the same time making it more difficult for governments to urge restraint in the use of resources.

Where do green ideas come from?

Green social and political thought emerged in the 1970s in response to the gathering alarm about finite resources and limits to growth. The ideas did not suddenly burst upon the world in the early 1970s, but have been around since the onset of industrialisation; what has changed is the accelerating impact of this process upon the natural world and our knowledge and understanding, through science, of the damage that is being wrought on our planet. Green ideas draw upon a variety of sources and are wide ranging in their scope, for they often start from the position that the damage done to the environment and nature stems from the deficient organisation of society and the economy, which means that this has to be rethought and in so doing non-statist and anarchist ideas have been utilised.

One source of green ideas in the UK was the nineteenth-century opposition to industrialisation and urbanisation. The filth, disease and poverty which was all too apparent in many of the industrial towns by the beginning of the nineteenth century produced a reaction among the new working class, who by the 1830s had slowly begun to organise themselves – albeit in small numbers – in trade unions and Chartism, the political movement which campaigned for the vote to be given to working men. Opposition also came from sections of the middle and upper class, and this is often characterised as the romantic critique of industrial capitalism. One of the most far-sighted critics of the new system was the writer John Ruskin (1819–1900). He reserved some of his most eloquent strictures for the economic system of production which reduced men and women to the status of 'hands' in mills and mines and he castigated industrial cities for their slums, which he asserted were an inevitable part of a system predicated upon greed. This critique was taken up, expanded and elaborated by the designer William Morris (1834–1896), who, in his socialist propaganda and notably in his book *News from Nowhere* (Morris, 1890), produced a powerful picture of a Britain after a socialist revolution where the cities had been deserted with the population living happily in the countryside. Until the end of the nineteenth century, sections of the working class still held to the idea that they would be able to move back to the countryside and, in the words of a political slogan used by the Liberal Party, have 'three acres and a cow'. This 'back to the land' movement came to nothing, producing little land for working people, and so was a failure in its own terms, although the introduction of allotments – land set aside specifically for the cultivation of fruit and vegetables in urban areas – was one result.

This nineteenth-century tradition had an abiding hatred of the squalor produced by city life and a corresponding idealisation of country life. Urbanisation was sufficiently novel for many people to think that the process could be reversed and that the nation could return to life in villages and small towns. This would be one solution to the high levels of unemployment in urban areas, which had led some to conclude that they were overpopulated.

Population

The concern over the size of the world's population dates back to the onset of industrialisation, and contemporary green thought is much exercised by the challenge posed by the dramatic rise in world population which threatens both the future of humanity and the natural resources upon which it depends. The English philosopher Thomas Malthus (1766–1834) was extremely influential at the beginning of the nineteenth century with his formulation that the rate of increase in population will always exceed the food resources. In his book *An Essay on the Principle of Population* – first published in 1798 – he maintained that any attempt to raise the standard of living of the poorest section of the population above subsistence was bound to end in failure because it would result in an increase in population with a consequent shortage of food (Malthus, 1970). At that time in the UK, unlike many European countries, there was a Poor Law, which would provide relief and assistance for those people who were destitute and had no other means of support. But Malthus argued that the Poor Law was encouraging people to enter into marriage when they could not afford the cost of bringing up children because they knew very well that if they were to get into financial difficulties the Poor Law would assist them. Malthus proposed that no one born after a certain date would be able to receive poor relief. This would enable the population increase to be curbed, which could be done most effectively by letting nature take its course, i.e. by allowing starvation and famine to remove excess population. Malthus believed that there were natural limits to population size – a view that many people would subscribe to today, although there are only a small minority who would agree with his methods for reducing population (Himmelfarb, 1984; Bramwell, 1989).

Darwin

Charles Darwin (1809–82), in his evolutionary work, accepted the Malthusian view of the shortage of resources. Human beings had to be seen as just one species: variations in individuals were passed on via those who succeeded in the struggle for survival. The 'fittest' were those who were most likely to survive, whereas those who were poorly adapted were likely to die out. As Pepper (1996: 183–4) remarks, Darwin's legacy for ecology supports both the idea of the dominance of humans over nature and a more benign view of co-existence between humans and nature where a 'brotherhood of creatures' participates in a co-operative scheme descending from common origins. In the 1860s, Ernest Haeckel (1834–1919) coined the term 'ecology' to refer to the science of relations between organisms and the environment, i.e. how species adapt to changes in the environment and the exchange of matter and energy between inter-related species of animals and plants (Harper, 1996: 12).

Contemporary green thought

As we saw in Chapter 1, the ecological perspective came to public attention in the early 1970s with the publication of landmark reports on the environment and the creation of the new green pressure groups such as Greenpeace and Friends of the Earth, responding to the growing evidence of the damage done to the environment by the industrial system. In Germany in the late 1970s, the Green Party (*Die Grunen*) was formed. This has been the most popular green political party and came out of an alliance between anti-nuclear power activists, the movement against nuclear weapons and the women's movement. (The UK Green Party has been hindered by the first-past-the-post electoral system, which has meant that it has not succeeded in getting a Member of Parliament elected to the Westminster parliament. Elections in this country for the European Parliament are held under the proportional representation system, and this has resulted in some British Green Members of the European Parliament.) Although *Die Grunen* was not the first green party, it has been the most influential in the formulation of an explicitly green perspective on politics and society.

Green thought was characterised from early on as 'neither left nor right', and this does capture an important aspect of the ecological/green perspective, i.e. the issues about which they are talking are not conventional party political ones. Everything else is seen in relation to the environment. With the environment as the guiding principle then the following principles are adhered to:

- Respect for nature and life forms.
- Respect for non-human life forms – this can take the form of vegetarianism or veganism or animal liberation.

- Commitment to treading lightly on the earth – trying to avoid those technologies such as planes or cars which damage the planet.
- Scepticism as to the claims of science and technology.
- Commitment to living simply and aversion to consumerism.

At least some of these themes are shared by greens of various persuasions, but the way in which they approach them varies considerably. We can say that there is a spectrum, with dark green being the most extreme to the lightest green.

Dark greens

Dark greens are those who are the most disenchanted with modern civilisation, blaming it for many of the woes which afflict the earth. They adopt an *ecocentric* approach, which prioritises nature over humankind. Because it is human beings who are causing the problems for the planet, this means that their numbers have to be reduced. Some writers, such as the American biologist Garret Hardin, believe that starvation is a natural occurrence and is just an illustration of nature keeping numbers in check, and therefore it would be unnatural to do anything about it. Human beings are taking far too much of the energy, resources and living space which they have to share with other creatures. The population question is the most important example of placing restrictions on individuals to protect nature. The dark-green view often involves the belief that rights to have children should be curtailed. Garret Hardin is the Malthus of our time. He wrote an extremely influential essay in 1968 entitled 'The Tragedy of the Commons' (Hardin, 1968) (Box 4.1). In another essay, he uses the metaphor of the rich world being akin to a full lifeboat surrounded by drowning swimmers (the poor world) (Hardin, 1977, cited in Pepper, 1996: 97) – should any of the swimmers be taken aboard when it is known that by this action the boat will sink? In Hardin's view, the problems caused by the right to reproduce freely are compounded by the commitment to universal human rights, for this can lead to more selfish behaviour which will further damage the environment. Furthermore, the pervasive belief in the capitalist economic system that individuals and societies can gradually increase their wealth and

Box 4.1 'The Tragedy of the Commons'

Picture a pasture open to all. It is to be expected that each herdsman will try to keep as many cattle as possible on the commons. Such an arrangement may work reasonably satisfactorily for centuries because tribal wars, poaching and disease keep the numbers of both man and beast well below the carrying capacity of the land. Finally, however, comes the day of reckoning, that is, the day when the long-desired goal of social stability becomes a reality. At this point the inherent tragedy of the commons generates tragedy.

As a rational being each herdsman seeks to maximise his gain. Explicitly, or implicitly, more or less consciously, he asks 'What is the utility to *me* of adding one more animal to my herd?' This utility has one negative and one positive component.

1   The positive component is a function of the increment of one animal. Since the herdsman receives all the proceeds from the sale of the additional animal, the positive utility is nearly +1.
2   The negative component is a function of the additional overgrazing created by one more animal. Since, however, the effects of overgrazing are shared by all the herdsmen, the negative utility for any one particular decision-making herdsman is only a fraction of −1.

Adding together the component partial utilities the rational herdsman concludes that the only sensible course for him to pursue is to add another animal to his herd. And another … and another. But this is the conclusion reached by each and every herdsman sharing a commons. Therein is the tragedy. Each man is locked into a system that compels him to increase his herd without limit − in a world that is limited. Ruin is the destination towards which all men rush, each pursuing his own best interest in a society that believes in the freedom of the commons. Freedom in a commons brings ruin to all.

(Hardin, 1968, cited in Daly, 1980)

consumption will also lead to an environmental collapse. The individuals and groups who pursue the 'good life' of consumerism are damaging the environment, but so too are the supporters of equal opportunities, universal health care and all the activities of the welfare state.

Just as for Malthus it was the Poor Law which was the villain because it kept poor people alive instead of allowing them to starve to death, so for Hardin it is the 'welfare state' which prevents nature taking its course. Hardin believes that it is only through the abandonment of the 'freedom to breed' that the planet has a chance of survival as a home for human beings. He uses the term 'carrying capacity' to refer to the ability of the planet to cope with its present numbers without degrading the environment. Yet we must remember that there are many who adhere to the deep-green viewpoint who find Hardin's views repugnant.

The deep-green philosophy entails an identification with a much wider self than the individualistic self of consumerism – it is a self which embraces nature and the organic webs in which every living creature is enmeshed on the planet. People should learn to feel part of the nature that is all around them, learning the features and contours of the area in which they live and in which they should remain (Devall, 1990; Dryzek, 1997: 156–8). This means appreciating the birds, trees, the habitat, the fauna and the flora where people live and being sensitive to the rhythms of nature, the light and dark provided by day and night, to enjoy the sensation of being out in the rain, the beauty of birds singing. Deep ecologists believe that these manifestations of nature are beautiful in themselves and this should make us pause for thought as to what we are doing to nature.

Although for deep ecologists it is human beings who are the problem, they do not mean all the world's human population, for they applaud the way in which some traditional societies live in harmony with nature – hunting, gathering, living on what is little more than a subsistence income. No, the people who are the problem are those living in the affluent countries of the world who use enormous amounts of energy each day and demand consumer goods, devastating nature because of the seemingly insatiable demand for natural resources. For the eight basic principles of deep ecology, see Box 4.2.

> **Box 4.2 The eight basic principles of deep ecology**
>
> 1   The well-being and flourishing of human and non-human life on Earth have value in themselves. ...These values are independent of the usefulness of the non-human world for human purposes.
> 2   Richness and diversity of life forms contribute to the realisation of these values and are also values in themselves.
> 3   Humans have no right to reduce this richness and diversity except to satisfy *vital* needs.
> 4   The flourishing of human life and cultures is compatible with a substantial decrease of the human population. The flourishing of non-human life requires such a decrease.
> 5   Present human interference with the non-human world is excessive and the situation is rapidly worsening.
> 6   Policies must therefore be changed. These policies affect basic economic, technological and ideological structures. The resulting state of affairs will be deeply different from the present.
> 7   The ideological change is mainly that of appreciating life *quality* ... rather than adhering to an increasingly higher standard of living.
> 8   Those who subscribe to the foregoing points have an obligation directly or indirectly to try to implement the necessary changes.
>
> (Devall and Sessions, 1985, in Pepper, 1996)

Eco-socialism

Green Parties in Western Europe tend to be associated with the political left despite the fact that one of the slogans used by greens is that they are 'neither left nor right, but in front'. It is true that the best-known Green Party – *Die Grunen* in Germany – is of the left, being formed in the very late 1970s out of a coalition between anti-nuclear activists and the women's movement. It can be argued that the greens are heirs to the long tradition of utopian thought which – as in the work of William Morris, aptly described as the first eco-Marxist – posited a future society that would be the end-point of human endeavour. The difference is that, in contrast to the late nineteenth century when Morris was writing, we are conscious of the ecological catastrophe waiting to happen if the direction of the world's economy and production is not shifted towards sustainability. At the same time, the green position is that unless there is a changed economy and society then the problems produced by industrialisation will return.

Eco-socialism is a broad term which can refer to two positions: greens who are also socialists and socialists who are green. The two are different – they are not identical: there is a difference between red greens and green reds! Red greens are those who believe that the environmental crisis is the most important issue in contemporary politics but believe that socialist policies will be the major way to tackle it. Green reds are people who believe that the distribution of income, resources and opportunities in society still remains the key issue but have a commitment to environmental policies. To connect this with the present reality of contemporary politics in the UK, one has to point out that the ideological position of the Labour Party – green red – on the environment is best described as ecological (or environmental) modernisation, which we will discuss later in this chapter.

The German Greens evolved in the 1980s out of a battle between what were called the realists and the fundamentalists. The latter were the group that has gone furthest to merge the perspectives of ecology and socialism into a coherent political position. Their spokesman Rudolf Bahro articulated this red–green vision in a series of books and speeches in the 1980s (Bahro, 1982, 1986). Bahro declared that what made his position fundamentalist was that he believed that the basic attitudes in affluent countries are oriented towards possessions and must change. This had been fuelled by the expansion of capitalism over the last 200 years – the most aggressive economic system in world history. Bahro argued against the industrial system as such – whether it be capitalist or not – and advocated 'industrial disarmament'. He called military installations, nuclear industry, projects to extend the transport infrastructure, airports, motorways, etc. the 'big machine';

essentially, he was referring to what many have called the 'military–industrial complex'. For him, production had become an end in itself, and the interests of wage-earners were bound up with the self-destruction of civilisation. A future green government would invest funds in the alternative sector – what is now called the social economy – of co-operatives and neighbourhood enterprise. Echoing the 'back to the land' movement of a century ago, Bahro argued that people must live off the land, which means that they need to acquire it in some way. His vision was that in the future people would live in base communities – which would have a maximum population of 3,000 – and they would agree that although they would reproduce the food and other essentials they needed they would not expand. So, in addition to growing their own food, the base communities would make their own clothes, construct their own housing, provide education, all by their own labour. Base communities would then contribute to the wider expenditure needed for the national infrastructure – for transport, media, government. This red–green fusion has some similarities to the anarchist and social ecology positions (Bahro, 1982, 1986; Dobson, 2000).

The French writer André Gorz is another major ideologue of the red–green position. Gorz has been particularly influential with his writings on the nature of work in capitalist society in which he argues for a social wage 'which would be paid to individuals in return for their performance of an agreed amount of labour over the course of their lifetime' (Kenny and Little in George and Page, 1995: 285). He defines three categories of work. The first of these categories is *macrosocial* activity, i.e. all the work, much of it unpleasant, which needs to be done to keep society functioning. The second category is *microsocial* activity; this is what can be called self-maintenance, the work of cooking, cleaning and for some people looking after children. In affluent societies, those who can afford to do so often pay someone else to do these tasks for them – a trend that Gorz abhors. *Autonomous* activity is the third category; this is doing what really interests one in life and is much more important than the other spheres. Gorz has argued that economic reason – the dominance of macrosocial activity over the others – has extremely detrimental consequences in our society, condemning millions to long hours of work but little life satisfaction (Gorz, 1989). Both Gorz and Bahro started out their ideological careers as Marxists, but both of them came to see its limitations in the face of questions which Marx did not have to deal with.

Social ecology

Social ecology is the term that the American writer Murray Bookchin uses to describe his perspective on ecology and socialism – he uses the term to emphasise the social dimension which he believes to be missing from much green thinking. Bookchin has elaborated in a series of books a philosophy of eco-living which draws heavily upon anarchism. His answer to the accumulating problems of industrial society is a society of decentralised communities which rely on the local hinterland for their food and production. This is 'a confederal society based on the co-ordination of municipalities in a bottom-up system of administration as distinguished from the top-down rule of the nation state' (Bookchin, 1992, in Barry, 1999: 91). Control and self-government would be at the local level, but the communities would share some authority for the maintenance of some national services with other communities around the country. Bookchin does not believe that the agents for this kind of new society will be the working class but rather new social movements such as the greens, feminists and the peace movement. It is not society as such which is to blame for the ecological problems which beset humankind but rather the fact that some sections of society bear much more responsibility than other parts, e.g. the transnational corporation in the oil industry is more culpable than the ordinary individual. Hierarchy is the root cause of our problems in relating to nature and the environment and Bookchin sees capitalism as a subset of hierarchy. He wants a society where everyone has the ability to participate in the formation of social policy and feels that it is in this way that hierarchy will be dissolved. But, as has been remarked, it is not impossible to find hierarchical organisations which can live in harmony with nature – the monastery is one such example (Eckersley, 1992: 150).

Eco-feminism

Eco-feminists draw parallels between domination of women by men and domination of nature by mankind.

In the eco-feminist view, patriarchy – the domination of society and women by men as exemplified in the male as breadwinner and the woman as mother and carer – assigned a place for women in the formula God–Man–Nature–Woman. Patriarchy emphasised the intuitive identification of women with nature, as expressed in their biology, which gave them special insights that men did not possess. The experience of pregnancy, childbirth and breast-feeding in particular made them much closer to nature. Nature was there to be dominated and made to serve the interests of man. Eco-feminists regard the suffering and exploitation inflicted on nature by men as somewhat akin to the suffering and oppression experienced by women. Some eco-feminists would, indeed, argue that women are closer to nature because of their biology, and this means that although men might be able to reason their way to an eco-feminist position they will never be able to *feel* it. In other words, women have a special insight into nature which men do not possess. Others would fiercely contest this view, for they feel that it plays into the hands of conservatives who wish to keep women out of the male worlds of work and power, instead confining them to home-making, child care and domesticity. Arguments that women are more virtuous than men can cut both ways, for they can be used to deny women access to the worlds of business and politics. This is only one eco-feminist position, however, and there are eco-feminists who link women's oppression and the exploitation of nature to a structural analysis of power in society. Usually, this is allied with a politics which emphasises that there needs to be a non-dominating and non-instrumental approach to nature. Another eco-feminist perspective comes from women in the poor world who argue that in their countries the culture does assign a high value to traditional female tasks and who defend women-based subsistence economies (Mellor, 1997: Ch. 3).

Green Conservatism

After Margaret Thatcher assumed the leadership of the British

Conservative Party in 1975, the majority of the party embraced a popular form of economic liberalism which emphasised the values of the market and individual freedom. This was not traditional conservatism, which had always seen a rightful place for the state and non-market forms of organisation. The words conservative and conservation share the same root, and Conservatives as the party of tradition had been the guarantors of features of English life such as commons, small villages and village life. This, after all, was the rural constituency which played so large a part in the continuing electoral success of the Conservatives in the twentieth century. John Gray (1993) has argued that the state and market forces between them have begun to undo the fabric of English life. Economic liberals argue that the market must be allowed to take its course. Take a regularly recurring conflict in local politics over the last two decades: a supermarket chain wants to build a superstore outside a county town and the local people are united in their opposition to this development for they know that it will close small shops and drain the life blood from their High Street. If the government decides for a variety of reasons – including free competition and the play of market forces – that the planning application should succeed, then what is happening here is the state favouring one form of capitalism over another and the green conservative view would be that it is small business which should be protected. Traditional conservativism accorded importance to tradition, order and prudence. An interesting development in the 1990s was the alliance formed in some English shires between traditional conservatives and eco-activists protesting against new road building.

There is no distinct tendency within the Conservative Party which has the label Green Conservative, but it is nonetheless a component of the traditional conservatism which used to be in the ascendancy in the Party.

The ideas that have been examined in this chapter so far have, to a greater or lesser extent, been utopian, concerned with some future society in which there will be harmony between humans and nature. For many years, greens were excellent at articulating the green society of the future, but were silent as to the means by which this new society would come about. This is much less the case now and the change can be attributed to two main reasons.

The Earth Summit in 1992 held in Rio de Janeiro put sustainable development on the world agenda and this has spawned a great deal of work on green policies and practice – most of it concerning the here and now. Around the same time, a number of mainstream thinkers across the political spectrum gave their attention to ecological issues; this was to some extent stimulated by Rio, although this work had started before the Earth Summit of 1992. In the rich world, the most influential corpus of ideas to come out of this encounter between mainstream thought and the environmental crisis is 'ecological modernisation'.

Ecological modernisation

Ecological modernisation differs from the ideologies that we have examined in this chapter so far in that it does not postulate a society in the future but instead believes that certain policies and certain ways of managing the economy will enable capitalist society to survive. Modernisation is required to make the economy environmentally responsive. Traditionally, it was thought that there was a natural opposition between environmental protection and economic growth. Ecological modernisation challenges this by claiming that the amount of energy used in the economy today is no more than it was 20 years ago, despite the increase in productivity and economic activity, because the energy used is utilised more productively. The ecological modernisation case is that we could be producing goods more efficiently with less energy. In addition, the process of pollution abatement and control yields economic rewards to those countries that have the latest technology and are able then to market it to the rest of the world.

Ecological modernisation seeks to back those industries which combine good economic returns with low environmental damage. At the same time, changes in the infrastructure mean that less energy is used because of changes in public transport, greater use of information technology and so forth. Building upon the insights generated by Weizsacker and colleagues, who argue that it is now possible to extract four times as much wealth from the resources that we use than in the past, it is argued that the technology is available for cars that will cross Europe on less than a gallon of petrol, for fridges that use half as much power as normal and windows that will let in light but block all outgoing heat and so on (Weizsacker *et al.*, 1997).

It can be seen that ecological modernisation goes with the grain of contemporary economic developments. In a global economy where manufacturing industry has migrated from the rich world to the poor world, then, naturally, pollution has reduced in the rich world. A service-led knowledge economy is going to be less damaging to the environment than one built around manufacturing industry. Ecological modernisers see the attraction of consumer capitalism but would want to encourage a more environmentally friendly consumption. They assign a central role to science and technology for the mastering of environmental problems.

Green futures

Environmental and green thinking is beginning to impinge on the practicality of government efforts to grapple with social and economic problems. The 1970s and 1980s were distinguished by the politics of protest for greens, whereas in the 1990s there has been much more of an engagement with contemporary political questions. As Barry (1999) has remarked, green political thought has moved on from the outlining of future green societies to proposing policies and solutions to contemporary social and environmental problems. Ecological modernisation has an obvious appeal to political elites because it does not presage a rupture with the contemporary pursuit of economic growth – it is the acceptable face of green thinking. In contrast to other green ideas, it is top-down in its policy implementation and does not require extensive participation by the citizenry.

The utopian greens – dark greens and eco-anarchists together with some eco-socialists – picture a future society in which relations between human beings and their relations with animals and the natural world have been radically altered to prevent exploitation and domination of nature. But this thinking does not have a strong purchase upon contemporary social policy, which inevitably has to be concerned with the here and now of social problems. In the next chapters, we will examine some of the ways in which green ideas are being applied in health, housing, food and work.

Key points

- Green ideas in the UK have their origin in the romantic critique of industrialism articulated by Ruskin and Morris together with the emergence of ecology in the nineteenth century.
- Dark greens and deep ecologists prioritise nature over humankind and advocate radical measures to curb human numbers and enable the population to live in harmony with nature.
- Eco-socialists are united in their belief that environmental problems are, in the main, caused by the capitalist economic system but differ in their solutions.
- Ecological modernisation is an attractive option for governments as it does not entail a break with existing policies on the economy and society but instead allows government to use its powers to steer the economy in a more sustainable direction.

Guide to further reading

Connelly, J. and Smith, G. (1999) *Politics and the Environment: From Theory to Practice*, London: Routledge. Thorough introduction to green thought and politics.

Dryzek, J.S. and Schlosberg, D. (eds) (1998) *Debating the Earth: The Environmental Politics Reader*, Oxford: Oxford University Press. Comprehensive collection of readings which covers all the main green positions.

Pepper, D. (1996) *Modern Environmentalism*, London: Routledge. Detailed account of the origins of contemporary environmental movement.

Smith, M.J. (ed.) (1999) *Thinking Through the Environment: a Reader*, London: Routledge. Key readings on intergenerational justice, animal welfare and ecological citizenship.

Chapter 5
Environmental health

Outline

Contemporary environmental problems stem from the organisation of industrial society. This chapter examines how this has produced a series of social policy responses and summarises the evidence on the links between health and air quality, transport emissions, water pollution and indoor pollution. The responses of government to the accumulating evidence on the dangers to public and individual health from environmental problems are outlined.

The relationship between the natural environment and health

When we carefully apply sun-tan lotion before going out on a sunny day, the link between 'the environment' and health is all too clear. The intensity of the sun caused by the thinning of the ozone layer is not something that we can easily ignore given the evidence of the increasing incidence of skin cancer. The consequences for the nation's health of the depletion of ozone is but one example of the impact of the environment upon our health. Climate change is a major hazard for humanity, calling into question our systems of industry, agriculture, fishing and food production. Although it is difficult to predict how – and in which direction – the climate will change and with what results, a change in disease patterns world-wide seems to be a likely result (McMichael, 1993) (Box 5.1). The impact of global warming on health in the UK was the subject of a 1992 report by the government's Public Health Laboratory. It

---

Box 5.1 **Main effects of global climate change on population health**

Direct
Deaths, illness and injury due to increased exposure to heat waves
Effects upon respiratory system
Climate-related disasters (cyclones, floods, fires, etc.)

Indirect
Altered spread and transmission of vector-borne diseases (cholera, influenza, etc.)
Disturbance and impairment of crop production – effects on soil, temperature, water, pests
Various consequences of sea level rise – inundation, sewage disruption, soil salinity, etc.
Demographic disruption, environmental refugees
(from McMichael, 1993: 144)

---

concluded that this would include the reintroduction of permanent endemic plague foci among rural rat populations; the arrival of the heart worm in Britain; an explosion in cockroach numbers with attendant health problems; and an increase in domestic mites (see Tindale, 1996). Malaria may well reappear in the UK – it was a permanent feature in the Middle Ages – with malarial insects having travelled in long-distance planes being able to survive in the warmer climate and then breed in this country (Brown, 1998). From even before the moment of conception our health is influenced by our environment, and to a greater or lesser extent all the topics covered in the following chapters – housing, food, employment – have an impact on the health of the population. Because of the extraordinary advances made by science and technology over the last century, it is arguable that nature no longer exists independently of humanity – it has been subordinated to human purposes (McKibben, 1990). The achievements of modern civilisation depend upon the use of the raw materials of nature: water, wood, coal, oil and gas have all been harnessed to create industrial societies. These processes can also be harmful to human health: chemicals released into rivers, pollutants which occur because of certain industrial processes, pesticides which get into our food.

This chapter examines the emergence of public health policy in the nineteenth century before assessing the contemporary impact of urbanisation on health. It reviews the health risks from environmental damage and the impact of air pollution, indoor pollutants and water pollution together with the health damage caused by motor transport. The chapter ends with a discussion of the way in which central government has moved towards the integration of environmental and health policy. As we shall see, the environmental health problems require the state to respond via the mechanisms of regulation and policy across a range of policy areas and not just healthcare.

The health consequences of industrialisation

The Industrial Revolution produced an array of health problems resulting from manufacturing and mining – diseases of the lungs, injuries from the new machinery and industrial diseases of many kinds. Workers lived close to the factories in mean streets, where disease spread rapidly, in cramped, overcrowded conditions without a clean water supply and with insufficient fruit and vegetables in their diet. The accumulated filth, sewage and pollution of the atmosphere created ideal conditions for the major killers – cholera, typhoid, diphtheria and tuberculosis. Charles Webster has described the Victorian inner cities as 'ecological disaster areas'. He writes 'In such districts mortality rates were often in the region of 40 per thousand population, while half the infants born died before the age of 5. These rates represent higher mortality levels than currently experienced in some of the most deprived third-world countries' (Webster, 1990: 5).

Local administration was designed for an earlier preindustrial age. The shaky administrative structures to be found in nineteenth-century towns and cities could not cope with the problems of overcrowding, disease and poor housing. Gradually, however, the nineteenth-century state came to regard public health as a matter of sufficient importance for it to intervene by means of regulation and policy. Government introduced legislation to promote the use of clean water supplies, the clearance of nuisances and the prosecution of polluters. Slowly, the health of the nation improved, as reflected in the infant mortality rate, crude death rates and patterns of sickness. The focus was on the health of the individual and how this was affected by the wider environment.

Since the mid-nineteenth century, there has been a realisation of the link between the environment and health which led to the introduction of piped water in Victorian cities from the middle of the nineteenth century, the employment of medical officers of health, the creation of the school medical service and a growth in public health activity by local authorities and central government. A public health profession emerged, with each local authority establishing a public health department headed by a medical officer of health with direct responsibility for the public health of citizens. The twentieth century saw unprecedented improvements in infant mortality rates, maternal mortality and life expectancy to name but some of the health indicators. This occurred before the introduction of antibiotics in the 1940s and was a result of higher wages, improved nutrition, better (and less insanitary) housing and slum clearance – in short, social policy was producing a better environment, which in turn led to healthier people. Today, environmental health officers employed by the local authority are responsible for food safety, control of vermin and a range of functions which can affect the general health of a neighbourhood. Although the title of Medical Officer of Health no longer exists, the work is performed by the public health staff of the health authority.

There is now a 'new public health' movement. While nineteenth-century public health concentrated on the physical environment, the 'new public health' concerns itself with the socioeconomic environment and prioritises environmental issues (Draper, 1991: 10).

This 'new public health' acknowledges the importance of a good diet, adequate housing, sufficient income, good education, clean air and water as well as an overall commitment to tackle social inequality. It is reflected to a certain extent in the government's decision that all health authorities should produce programmes to improve the health of the population by working in co-operation with the local authority and other agencies. The new public health perspective can also be seen in the programmes to improve the health of city dwellers in the contemporary world.

Urban health

Urbanisation continues apace in the contemporary world, producing pressing health problems. The barrios of Latin America and the shanties of Africa and Asia are eloquent testimony to the appeal of urban life for the landless people who migrate from rural areas. They are the most visible sign of the incapacity of the urban system to cope with the demands placed upon it. The promulgation of the attractions of Western consumerism to the people of the poor world via television, with its glorification of the lifestyles of the rich, means that millions aspire to this way of life, and economic migration is one result. Migration from rural to urban areas in search of work is a long-established phenomenon, whereas the international migration from poor countries to rich countries has been made easier by modern forms of transportation. The development of modern cities introduced new hazards to health, such as traffic accidents, the rapid spread of infection, homelessness and poverty wages. The massing of populations in the cities of the poor world means that airborne diseases spread quickly from person to person. Today, the most heavily populated cities in the world face acute problems of public health. Cairo has a population of 12 million, but its sewerage system was established when the city had a population of 2 million (McMichael, 1993: 267). The people in these new mega-cities of the poor world are also prone to the worst air pollution, with traffic and industrial fumes damaging their respiratory systems. Poor countries who do not have health and environmental regulations to protect their populations are an attractive location for some unscrupulous companies, resulting in exploitation of children's labour and overlong hours often worked in unsafe and unhygienic conditions.

Environmental risk

Environmental risks are a major worry. The greater awareness of the environmental components which lead to death and disease are sources of anxiety. People look to government to protect them against environmental risk but this is sometimes difficult when the rate of scientific innovation is so rapid. Risk has come to dominate the environmental agenda since the release of nuclear radiation with the nuclear accident at Chernobyl in the former Soviet Union in 1986. Nowadays, risk is high on the climatologists agenda as the world has been experiencing historically high temperatures, which would suggest that we are now beginning a period of climatic change.

Risk is a concept which has become very fashionable in the social sciences of late – one might say that it is an example of the social sciences mirroring the contemporary world and its preoccupations, for risk has become a topic of real interest in a world where so much that was previously thought of as fixed is now open to the possibility of change. Medical science has enabled many more people to enjoy a longer life and, indeed, to have a life – those who have genetic disorders which are now treatable or those who have organ transplants which enable them to live or to see. Arguably, the advances made by medical science in the preservation of human life are not always for the best – the carers of those with traumatic brain injury which has damaged their sensory, mental and locomotor abilities might sometimes feel that it would have been more humane for the doctors to allow the injured to die in the aftermath of the accident.

Yet, proportionality of risk is an important consideration – in any one year the risk of dying if one smokes ten cigarettes per day is 1:200, whereas the risk of dying in a road accident is 1:10,000 and from nuclear radiation is 1:10,000,000 (Porritt, 2000: 36).

The precautionary principle has been promoted by environmentalists: if there is an absence of clear-cut scientific proof, this cannot be used as an excuse to delay measures to safeguard the environment or human health if there is a risk of serious or irreversible harm. This was endorsed by the World Health Organization in its European Charter on Environment and Health, which states that 'New policies, technologies and developments should be introduced with prudence and not before appropriate prior assessment of the potential environmental and health impact. There should be a responsibility to show that they are not harmful to health or the environment' (see Crombie, 1995: 16).

The environmental risks to health often mainly affect those who are the most disadvantaged in society. Those who live in heavily trafficked streets, especially children and those with respiratory conditions, face a daily assault on their health. If they are on low incomes, then their chances of moving to a less polluted area are low.

Those people with superior financial resources use these to minimise risk to themselves and their families – they do not live in areas of industrial pollution or near busy main roads with high levels of traffic and their employment does not expose them to dangerous processes. Official advice on the best way to protect against risks to health often consists of health education messages – the government's promotion of eating fruit and vegetables is presented as reducing the risk of contracting cancer. Likewise, the encouragement to exercise is regarded as a means of keeping healthy. But air pollution is one example of an environmental health risk which at certain times is more likely to confront those who live on low incomes or in poor areas

Air pollution

Much of the pollution that is threatening to health cannot be seen; this is the case with a great deal of air pollution, and air quality has become an object of concern once again in recent years. In the nineteenth century and early twentieth century, the smogs which enveloped industrial towns were responsible for increased mortality rates and for the worsening of conditions such as respiratory illness. Gradually, action was taken to restrict and outlaw the pollution caused by coal emissions and coal-burning power stations. The last major outbreak of airborne pollution of this kind was the London smog in December 1952, which led to 4,700 deaths (Department of Health, 1997). Yet industrial pollution has not disappeared, although the use of coal is much less than it was a quarter of a century ago.

Health and pollution

The World Health Organization has estimated that millions of Europeans live in areas where they are exposed to unnecessarily high levels of pollutants. Principally, these are areas of central and Eastern Europe which were sites of heavy industry under their previous Communist governments (World Health Organization Regional Office for Europe, cited in Rowell *et al.*, 1992). Although Box 5.2 shows those groups in the population most at risk from air pollution, there are a host of intervening variables – age, sex, medical condition – which mean that susceptibility to pollutants varies considerably from one person to another.

Air pollution is known to aggravate respiratory and cardio-vascular illness and is believed to be a contributory factor in certain diseases and forms of cancer.

Industrial pollution

The emission of pollutants from factories and manufacturing plants is a major contributor to poor air quality. Industrial pollution does not fall impartially on rich and poor areas alike. A Friends of the

---

Box 5.2 The adverse health effects of air pollution

Those most at risk are:

- children under 5 years;
- children aged 5–14 years;
- people over 65 years;
- people with asthma;
- people with other respiratory conditions;
- people with cardiovascular conditions;
- unborn babies and pregnant women.

(from Rowell *et al.*, 1992)

Earth survey demonstrated that the more factories there are in a neighbourhood then the lower the income. Of the UK's largest factories, 662 are in areas where the average household income is less than £15,000 and only five are in areas where the average household income is £30,000 per year or more (Friends of the Earth, 1999). As Phillimore and Moffatt (1999) have shown in their work on industrial pollution on Teesside, there is a reluctance to admit to the degree of pollution in certain districts close to chemical plants and other processes. Understandably, the firms producing the pollution wish to minimise the risks to local people, while local authorities do not want to frighten away inward investment.

Clearly, there are historical reasons why there is a concentration of chemical plants and other environmentally hazardous factories in the Teesside area. Those who built the houses so close to the plants were probably unaware of the dangers to the health of the local people. It is a vivid example of what has been termed environmental injustice, where those living in deprived areas who already have to contend with poverty, high levels of crime and educational disadvantage also find their health affected by high levels of pollution. The connection between low-income areas and industrial pollution is not to be found uniformly across the UK, but it is a feature of some of the older industrial regions.

Transport pollution

The major hazard (Box 5.3) to the quality of our air in urban areas comes from transport and, in particular, the spectacular growth in the use of the private car. Two forms of pollution need to be distinguished: primary pollutants are those released directly into the air from cars, such as carbon monoxide, nitric oxide, benzene and particulates (the microscopic particles which are released into the air from the burning of diesel fuel), and secondary pollutants are formed by chemical changes to the primary pollutants, e.g. nitrogen dioxide is formed from nitric oxide while a photochemical process breaks down the nitrogen dioxide to produce ozone (Box 5.3).

Diesel engines are responsible for particulates, the tiny particles to be found in vehicle emissions, which cause approximately 8,000

Box 5.3 Health hazards from transport pollutants

Benzene: a cancer-causing aromatic hydrocarbon produced principally by vehicle exhausts and fuel evaporation.

Ozone: formed by chemical reactions involving nitrogen oxides and volatile organic compounds with around half of both coming from road transport. Ozone depletion, which produces increased ultraviolet light, will result in more cataracts and skin cancers.

1,3-Butadiene: a carcinogen arising mainly from vehicle exhausts.

Carbon monoxide: can impair brain function and cause headaches. Over 90 per cent is from road transport, with nearly 90 per cent of this from cars.

Sulphur dioxide: responsible for acid rain. Produced mainly by non-transport sources.

Particulates: aggravate respiratory diseases with possible other health impacts. About half comes from diesel-powered transport.

Nitrogen oxides: cause respiratory problems as well as contributing to the formation of ozone. About half come from road vehicles.

Lead: damages the blood, bone marrow and nervous system, and can affect kidney and brain function.

Polycyclic aromatic hydrocarbons: include known carcinogens and contained in petrol vapour.

Note: carbon dioxide does not have health effects, although it is the major 'greenhouse gas' contributing to global warming.

(Crombie, 1995; Potter, 1997: 31)

excess deaths each year in the UK. They damage the lung and are believed to cause tumours (Department of Health, 1999). A report by the Department of Health Committee on the Medical Effects of Air Pollutants (1997: 98) stated 'Most authorities now accept that the case for a relationship between mass concentrations of particles and effects on health is compelling'. Car drivers face pollution levels from particulates in their car which are two to three times higher than those experienced by pedestrians (Department of the Environment, Transport and the Regions, 1998b: 2.8). The government believes that levels of particulates need to be progressively reduced, but this is not a straightforward task given that the number of cars in the UK continues to increase year by year. Benzene is another hazard because of its widespread dispersion by motor vehicles. Its presence in petrol means that it is a daily hazard to millions of people. Benzene concentrations have been the subject of much research, and it is now accepted that it is a cancer-causing agent and there are no absolutely safe levels. The main sources of benzene are vehicle exhausts, petrol refining and emissions from petrol station forecourts. Benzene levels inside cars are higher than those in the ambient air outside the vehicle (Department of the Environment, Transport and the Regions, 1998b).

The government has an air quality strategy which states the safe levels for pollutants. This is done within the context set by the EU directives on air pollution. Local authorities have a duty to assess air quality in their areas, and if air quality is deemed to be poor then they have to produce plans to improve it. Health improvement programmes will be one of the mechanisms whereby the health authority and the local authority can work together to improve air quality (see p. 87).

Transport and health

The accumulating evidence on the extent to which vehicle emissions exacerbate existing medical conditions and, indeed, produce certain cancers and shorten life constitute part of the public health problem of transport. The impact of air pollution from transport, however, is overshadowed by the fear of serious injury or death, and this has most resonance when we travel on our roads or cross the road as a pedestrian. World-wide, road accidents kill or disable more people than tuberculosis, human immunodeficiency virus (HIV) or war each year. Since the first road death in 1896, cars have claimed 30 million lives. Currently, 500,000 people per year die and 15 million are injured (Tickell, 1998). Seventy per cent of road deaths now occur in developing countries – the result of the fact that cars are being driven on streets where there is still a considerable amount of walking and cycling. The Red Cross predicts that by 2020 road accidents will cause more deaths world-wide than tuberculosis, war and HIV (Brown, 1998) (see Box 5.4).

The global statistics on the annual toll of death and serious injury do not reveal the full extent of this health problem, for the health

---

Box 5.4 World Health Organization action plan for member states on transport, environment and health

- Integrate environment and health requirements and targets into transport policies.
- Promote modes of transport and land use planning which have best public health impacts.
- Conduct health and environment impact assessment of transport policies.
- Identify the economic costs of transport on the environment and health.
- Ensure special care of groups at extra risk of the negative health effects of transport.
- Research the risks for public health from transport, not yet quantified.
- Establish indicators and monitor progress made towards the targets identified.
- Promote pilot projects and research programmes into sustainable and healthy transport.
- Increase public participation, public awareness and information.

(from *Charter on Transport, Environment and Health*, WHO Europe, 1999; quoted in Hamer, 1999) costs extend to the friends and families of the victims who have been killed or seriously injured. A large proportion of the relatives of the dead or disabled suffer psychological problems. Anxiety attacks, suicidal feelings and depression are all commonly reported. There is a continuing cost to the health-care system in treatment and care for the injured. Head injuries occur in around half of road accidents, producing neurological disorders, loss of memory, inability to perform normal tasks and an inability to concentrate (European Federation of Road Traffic Victims, 1997).

In the UK, some caution needs to be exercised with accident figures, for there is a degree of under-reporting – this applies particularly to pedestrian and cyclist accidents.

The considerable fall in the number of fatalities on the roads (Table 5.1) between 1977 and 1994 – a drop of 28 per cent – does not, unfortunately, mean that the roads are safer in the 1990s than in the 1970s. During that time the number of cars on the roads has more than doubled (Potter, 1997: 2).

Roads have become more dangerous, and this has meant that walking and cycling have declined as travel modes. This has had considerable impact for some road users, e.g. children are much more restricted in their ability to travel than in previous generations.

The transport systems of modern cities also make it more difficult for people to exercise their bodies – although public parks and open spaces are some compensation – and the costs of travelling to the countryside are often too high for the poor and the low paid to bear. Walking and cycling are both excellent forms of aerobic exercise, and if adopted by more people as a form of transport for short journeys then levels of physical fitness would improve.

Noise is another side-effect of the big increase in traffic on UK roads. 'Silence is becoming an increasingly scarce commodity in our towns and cities' (Maddison *et al.*, 1996: 84). The impact of noise on health is to be found in annoyance, sleep disturbance, heart disease and impaired performance in school children (Health Education Authority, 1998). The sources of noise can be seen in Table 5.2, which is derived from the National Noise Incidence Study.

The World Health Organization has formed an action plan for member states on transport, environment and health (Box 5.4).

Table 5.1 Transport accidents, 1977, 1987 and 1994

	1977		1987		1994		1987–94 (% change)	
	Killed	All severities	Killed	All severities	Killed	All severities	Killed	All severities
Road users								
Child pedestrians	440	30,374	245	19,934	160	19,263	−35	0
Child cyclists	95	9,705	68	7,934	42	8,075	−38	+2
Adult pedestrians	1,869	38,977	1,454	36,587	953	28,091	−34	−23
Adult cyclists	206	13,392	212	18,479	129	16,704	−39	−13
Motorcyclists	1,182	71,689	723	45,801	444	24,309	−39	−47
Car drivers and passengers	2,441	151,510	2,206	159,468	1,764	195,109	−20	+22
Light goods vehicle drivers and passengers	152	11,369	111	8,842	64	7,554	−42	−15
Heavy goods vehicle drivers and passengers	109	4,491	75	3,487	41	3,370	−45	−3
Bus/coach passengers and drivers	64	12,375	15	9,088	21	10,082	−40	+11
All road	6,558	343,882	5,109	309,620	3,650	315,189	−28	+2
Rail								
Railway passengers	27	1,778	36	2,689	12[a]	2,227[a]	−67	−17
Railway staff	28	395	11	85	3[a]	204[a]	−73	+140
Others	6	11	10	3	12[a]	13[a]	+20	[c]
All rail	61	2,184	57	2,777	27[a]	2,444[a]	−52	−12

Public air services

Passengers	2	2	0	1	0	2	–[c]	–[c]
Staff	9	2	1	5	1	2	–[c]	–[c]
Other air users[b]	20	43	53	56	27	38	–49	–32
All air	31	47	54	63	22	38	–59	–40
Total	6,650	346,113	5,219	312,460	3,705	317,675	–29	+2

Source: Potter (1997: 43).

Notes

a Financial year 1994/5.

b Executive, clubs and private, etc.

c Figures too small to make a valid comparison.

Table 5.2 Noise sources outside dwellings, 1986–91

Noise source	Percentage main source	Percentage of sites recording source
Road traffic	66	93
Aircraft	3	31
Railways	1	14
Construction	1	4
Industry	1	2
People	13	73
Animals	2	38
Birds	4	8
Mowers	2	11
Wind	5	7

Source: Maddison *et al.* (1996: 85).

Water pollution

Water is a key resource for life on this planet. Human life is impossible without it, and the great majority of the world's diseases are attributable to a lack of a clean water supply. Outbreaks of hepatitis, cholera and typhoid thrive when there is a dirty water supply, and dirty water supports the flies that spread eye diseases such as trachoma in developing countries. Children and young people are particularly susceptible to these diseases. In the UK, we are favoured by the climate so we do not experience the serious droughts which affect some other countries, and this is perhaps one of the reasons why we might be said to be profligate in the use of water. During the last few decades, the use of water has increased considerably, stimulated by the spread in ownership of consumer products such as washing machines, dishwashers and the growth in popularity of the shower in private households. The privatisation of water companies has put the issue of water supply under the spotlight as companies increased charges in order to pay for essential work to improve the quality of the supply and to repair broken pipes which are causing waste of water.

With the world facing serious water shortages in the twenty-first century and the growing urbanisation of the planet leading to water shortage, then on environmental grounds the present UK system of providing water supply without reference to the amount used is clearly indefensible. Water metering is as sensible as electricity or gas metering. Fewer than 10 per cent of households in the UK have water meters, and in those areas where they do exist for domestic consumers there is evidence that they cause hardship for those on low incomes (McLaren *et al.*, 1998: 196). Huby (1998: 56) points out that:

> A recent report on the impact of metering on low-income families found that although 70 per cent were taking measures to reduce their use of water, these measures were mainly limited to sharing baths or bathing less frequently, washing clothes less often, flushing the lavatory less often and preventing children from playing with water.

The quality of the bathing water on the coastline is a health hazard. The dumping of raw sewage has reached a point where the sea cannot cope with this and still provide clean water for bathing. Twenty-six billion litres of sewage are produced every day in the UK and 1.4 billion litres are discharged untreated into the sea. Of the seventy-two towns and cities pumping untreated sewage in the EU countries, twenty-two of them are in the UK (European Commission, 2001; Marine Conservation Society, 2001). The result is that bathing in the water off many of Britain's beaches presents a health hazard and people who swim in sea waters are more likely to suffer from infections and illness. One-fifth of our beaches were below EU standards when tested for most bacteria (Friends of the Earth, 1998b).

Indoor pollutants

Indoor pollutants are of great importance in our lives simply because most of us spend 80 per cent of our time indoors – whether at home or at work. One of the most dangerous pollutants is cigarette smoking, which is a direct cause of most lung cancer and is responsible for one-third of all deaths from cancer (Department of Health, 1999). There has been growing concern not only about the risk to smokers themselves but also to those who passively inhale the nicotine. This is especially dangerous for children as they have immature respiratory systems. 'Children of parents who smoke inhale the same amount of nicotine as if they themselves smoked 60–150 cigarettes a year' (Rosenbaum, 1993: 72). Cooking and heating systems can generate pollutants: carbon monoxide poisoning, for example, accounts for around 100 deaths per year. Radon, a natural gas released from small quantities of uranium that seeps out of the ground, house dust mites and nitrogen dioxide are also sources of pollution indoors (British Medical Association, 1998: 108).

Healthy cities

The World Health Organization's 'Healthy Cities' project aims to make sure that health is a high priority for decision-makers and works with disadvantaged groups to improve their health status and environment. Behind the idea of the 'Healthy City' lie two dominant perspectives which are sometimes in conflict: healthy lifestyles and an improvement in the environment.

> Cities should, according to the Health Cities philosophy, provide a clean and safe physical environment of a high quality based upon suitable eco-systems. They should offer their inhabitants access to the prerequisites for health (food, income, shelter) – and a wide variety of experiences based upon a diverse, vital and innovative economy.
> (Tsouros and Draper in Davies and Kelly, 1993: 25–6)

Healthy cities are not those which have achieved a certain level of health for their citizens, rather they are cities that are conscious of health and that intend to improve the health of the city. In the UK, they are the London Borough of Camden, Liverpool, Glasgow and Belfast. Healthy cities projects in the UK work closely with Local Agenda 21, and as we shall see many of the themes are now promoted by central government as part of their public health strategy.

The Ottawa Charter of the World Health Organization in 1986 spoke of the need to achieve healthy public policies and a supportive environment to underpin health. In Frankfurt in 1989, the World Health Organization published its *European Charter on Environment and Health*. The charter declared that 'every individual is entitled to an environment conducive to health. Every individual also shares the responsibility for securing good health within the environment and cannot merely depend on others for protection' (WHO, 1989: 29). Each person must regard it as their obligation to care for the environment in order to secure it as a healthy environment. The Ottawa Charter stated that:

> Our societies are complex and interrelated. Health cannot be separated from other goals. The inextricable links between people and their environments constitute the basis for a socio-ecological approach to health. The overall guiding principle for the world, nations, regions and communities alike, is the need to encourage reciprocal maintenance – to take care of each other, our communities and our natural environment. The conservation of natural resources throughout the world should be emphasised as a global responsibility.
>
> (cited in Jones and Sidell, 1997: 193)

In 1994, the Helsinki Declaration on Action for Environment and Health in Europe was launched, resulting in European National Environmental Health Action Plans. By 1998, over 90 per cent of EU member states had developed these plans. In 1999, the Third Ministerial Conference on Environment and Health held in London voiced concerns on a wide spectrum of health issues related to environmental problems and debated ways in which concrete local and national action can improve health conditions in Europe. A parallel non-governmental organisation (NGO) event (the Healthy Planet) enabled NGOs, local authorities and academics to formulate positions on issues discussed at the ministerial conference. The following areas provide examples of the Ministerial conference recommendations and reveal how closely environment and health were linked.

The first of these is a charter on transport, environment and health, including a proposal for an integrated European rail network and outlining specific measures such as health and environmental impact assessment of traffic to quantify public health hazards. Ministers agreed a declaration to establish four areas of national policy that damage children's health: tobacco smoke, food production, distribution and consumption. They did not specifically address inequalities but drew attention to the increasing inequity between and within countries. In the Ministerial declaration, countries committed themselves to working together on five research areas: water quality, air quality, environmental effects on cognitive functions, unintentional injuries to children and climate change.

The health promotion staff employed by the National Health Service (NHS) focus on the important role that can be played by local people in the determination of priorities for their area. Increasingly, they are adopting a new public health agenda; much of the work of the health promotion staff employed by the NHS could be said to be environmental – promoting cycling, walking, healthy foods – and the local Friends of the Earth group will often have a similar agenda.

New Labour, health and the environment

Following the Rio Summit of 1992 and the new commitment to sustainable development in health policy, it was in the areas of public and environmental health that government concentrated its attention. In 1996, *The United Kingdom National Environmental Health Action Plan* was published (Department of Health, 1996). Like so much government policy in this area, it reiterated the action that was already being taken by the government, describing the contribution of local authorities, the Health and Safety Executive and other bodies. There was the familiar consensual embrace: 'The government has always recognised that the task of achieving sustainable development involves the whole country – central and local government, business, other organisations and individuals. Ultimately it depends upon the choices about their lifestyles made by each member of society' (Department of Health, 1996: 1, 7). It emphasised that lifestyle choice is clearly important: personal decisions can be made regarding smoking, eating and exercise and there is a large of information around about this. Although this is undoubtedly true, we all make choices within a context and for some people this context is one where they have adequate leisure, low stress levels, a good income, an interesting job and a warm and supportive family. For too many people, however, that context is one of poverty, in which there is never enough income to satisfy their aspirations, where their housing is poor, they have no car and public transport is expensive and unreliable.

The Conservative government's major intervention in public health was *The Health of the Nation* strategy published in 1992, which committed the NHS to reaching targets in the reduction of accidents, heart disease and stroke, cancer, mental illness, HIV/ AIDS and sexual health. Towards the end of the Major government, the environment was adopted as one of the key areas for that strategy. The Labour government elected in 1997 outlined its approach in *Our Healthier Nation*, which declared that one of its key aims was 'to improve the health of the worst off in society and to narrow the health gap' (Department of Health, 1998a: 5). Among the factors affecting health (see Table 5.3), this document listed 'environmental factors', and these included air quality, housing, water quality and social environment. The last phrase, 'social environment', is defined in the document in the following way: 'The quality of life in the community and the extent to which people respect and support each other can also be important to our health'. This accords with the stress in New Labour thinking on the revival of community and neighbourhood development. The government pledged that they 'will ensure that the influence of the environment on health is fully recognised and integrated into major policy

Table 5.3 Factors affecting health

Fixed	Social/economic	Environment	Lifestyle	Access to services
Genes	Poverty	Air quality	Diet	Education
Sex	Employment	Housing	Physical activity	NHS
Ageing	Social exclusion	Water quality	Smoking	Social services
		Social environment	Sex/drugs	Leisure

Source: Department of Health (1998a).

initiatives, particularly in the sustainable development strategy, and in the transport strategy' (Department of Health, 1998a: 3.32).

A problem for any government is that environmental imperatives and individuals' preferences for their lives can come into conflict. For obvious reasons, politicians do not want unduly to antagonise their electorate and this can lead them to soften environmental policies. People brought up on the imperatives of consumerism may react badly when they are told to cut back on their levels of buying and spending, especially as the dominant messages of the mass media and advertising assume a high-consumption lifestyle. The antennae of modern politicians – focus groups and other market research techniques – are quick to pick up on these negative reactions and will modify policies accordingly. It is not the case that all other policy considerations are subordinated to environmental imperatives. Political parties, whether in government or opposition, are extremely sensitive to public opinion and are sophisticated enough to realise that the environmental noises we make when confronted with a clipboard in the High Street are not necessarily the personal preferences that we manifest in what we buy or how we travel. Within government, environmental policies have to fight for attention and support and are often simply not given sufficient priority because they do not have the weight or the more immediate appeal of employment policy, education or health care. Environmental issues are often more intangible and less obvious in their impact on individuals. We have to take government pronouncements with some caution for they represent aspirations in a keenly fought policy arena in which environment is just one of a number of policies. A welcome innovation has been the emphasis on policy linkage – or 'joined-up government' – meaning that, for example, transport documents now carry a paragraph or two which point to the health policy implications of any suggested policy direction and recommend that local authorities and health authorities keep in close contact. This attempt at policy integration is mirrored at the local authority and local health authority levels, where policy documents stress the importance of joint working with other agencies in partnership.

Joint working between agencies – intersectoral co-operation – is destined to become more important with the implementation of health improvement programmes by all local health authorities. Health improvement programmes are an agreed statement of the most important health needs and health problems in each locality. *Our Healthier Nation* listed the environmental factors of air and water quality and housing, and it is expected by the government that local health authorities will work closely with local authorities, among others, on issues such as healthy transport policies and healthy food policies for the local population. Health improvement programmes are 3-year rolling programmes which assess the health needs of the area and how they can be met. These are to be co-ordinated by the local health authority in association with the local authority, the primary care groups (GPs and health workers in the community) and the local NHS trusts (the hospitals). They involve:

- an agreed statement of the most important health needs and problems locally;
- a commitment from all parties to share information and to work jointly to improve our knowledge of problems and how they can be tackled;
- a 3-year statement of agreed strategies and action by and between agencies to make improvements in health in the medium and long term;
- a framework for the service and financial arrangements in the NHS and between the NHS and social services.

They are a means whereby environmental issues which impinge upon the health of individuals and groups can be addressed, e.g. air quality and transport.

The commitment to tackling health inequality shown by the New Labour government has led to the creation of area-based strategies, and health action zones (HAZs) are among these. Health action zones are designed to:

- identify and address the public health needs of their areas and devise new ways of tackling health inequalities;
- modernise services by increasing their effectiveness and responsiveness.

There are twenty-six zones, and these cover more than 13 million people. They are located in those parts of the country which have the highest scores on indices of social deprivation. Here, too, there are opportunities for the linking of health and environmental policy as HAZs are designed as partnerships between local health authorities, local authorities, the voluntary and private sector and community groups. This is aided by the fact that they have the same boundaries as local authorities.

The Environment Agency has the responsibility for monitoring the quality of river water, ground water and coastal water. The Environment Agency is not a health organisation, but it is responsible for the regulation of certain areas which impinge upon human health, e.g. its responsibility for rivers and river water quality and its brief to improve air quality. The Agency was established by merging the National Rivers Authority and Her Majesty's Inspectorate of Pollution and started work in 1996. The principal responsibilities of the Environment Agency are:

- to regulate industrial processes to prevent or reduce pollution;
- to regulate the disposal of radioactive waste;
- to regulate the treatment, movement and disposal of controlled waste;
- to regulate contaminated land;
- to preserve or improve the quality of rivers;
- to conserve proper use of water resources;
- to supervise flood defence systems.

The British Medical Association (BMA) has said that the Environment Agency should acknowledge much more clearly than it has done to date the relationship 'between the health of the environment and the health of the population'. To this end, the BMA recommends that the Environment Agency appoints a medical officer in each region who would have the task of examining the consequences of environmental regulation for health (British Medical Association, 1998). Its 1998 strategy document identifies the prevention of harm to human health as one of its key functions in relation to waste.

Healthy social policy

The health of individuals is linked to the culture and values to be found within the society in which those individuals live. The Conservative government document on public health, *Our Healthier Nation*, referred to 'the social environment', i.e. the web of relationships and social interactions that surround us in society and are important for our health. Those societies with high levels of trust – where people have faith and confidence in one another and hence there are high rates of participation in voluntary organisations and other forms of communal activity – would appear to be healthier, i.e. they have lower levels of sickness and better mortality rates. Wilkinson (1996) and others have demonstrated that there is a relationship between income inequality rates in a country and average life expectancy. The more unequal a society is in its distribution of income and wealth then the worse its health statistics will be. To some extent this is because of the poverty that will result from a skewed distribution of resources in unequal societies, but authors such as Wilkinson (1996) claim that trust, reciprocity and good will are essential attributes of a healthy society. It is social capital which contributes to the health indices of a society, i.e. the degree to which there is a network of voluntary, informal and family organisations. There is accumulating evidence that inequality can affect people's sense of subjective well-being – poor conditions of public life with vandalism and high crime rates can have an impact on health status as well.

It can be argued that the unhealthiness of society is to be found in the predominant value system which emphasises the accumulation of material goods as constituting the meaning of life, i.e. consumerism. This leads to the engendering of feelings of dissatisfaction and deprivation relative to others. Robert H. Frank (1999) reports that in the USA conspicuous consumption spending, on luxury homes, luxury hotels, pleasure yachts, cosmetic surgery, designer clothing and expensive cars, is at a record high. He argues that this is driven by the insecurities that people have in a consumer society as to how they are faring in comparison with their peer group. The evidence now emerging is that in consumer societies such as the USA and the UK – where there is a high attachment to paid employment, long hours, status consumption – the health indicators are worse than those of societies where there is a high degree of trust and an active civil society. As Frank (1999: 175) points out, it is the inconspicuous consumption which does most for the health and sanity of a society, in other words time spent with friends and family, parks and open spaces, freedom from traffic congestion. But this is not reflected in the advertising on the mass media, which may be said to be a guide to the good life. People's subjective sense of their own well-being matters, and the high levels of depression, anxiety and stress in consumer societies such as our own contribute to increased ill-health and a poor social environment (James, 1997).

The association between feelings of well-being and good physical and mental health are now recognised, although the ways in which these connections occur are not completely understood. The pressures on people in advanced societies to consume are many and varied. The income needed for the enjoyment of foreign holidays, cars and all the other prerequisites for the 'good life' in a consumer society have meant that paid employment has marginalised other activities – the statistics on voluntary work show a decline, many people report less time spent with their friends and family – and, indeed, one of the stresses that many people complain of in modern life is lack of time. Young children are a very needy group of the population and they soak up lots of time. Yet in the consumer societies of the UK and the USA there has been a clear move away from mothers staying at home for the early years of their children's lives, with women increasingly going back into the workforce when their children are still at an early age. This has not been compensated for by fathers spending more time with their children to make up the deficit. There is some well-founded concern that because the first 2 years of a child's life are vital for the formation of secure attachments then the increased use of day care, nannies and nurseries by parents is leading to an increase in separation anxiety, with the possibility of resulting problems for the mental health of these children (James, 1997).

There can be no doubt that the environmental crisis which confronts the planet will lead to accumulating health problems. The twin processes of industrialisation and urbanisation which now have the entire world in their grip will further disrupt patterns of livelihood and produce continuing problems for public health. Human ingenuity combined with environmental awareness has the ability to improve further health care world-wide, but climatic change may well defeat humanity's resolve.

Key points

- Industrialisation and urbanisation combined with climate change dictate the context in which global health care can operate.
- Risks to human health pose considerable problems for societies which are undergoing rapid technological and societal change.
- Transport emissions have numerous health consequences.
- New Labour has begun the process of linking health and environmental issues.

Guide to further reading

British Medical Association (1998) *Health and Environmental Impact Assessment*, London: Earthscan. Sets out the case for an integrated approach to health and the environment.

Jones, L. and Siddell, M. (eds) (1997) *The Challenge of Promoting Health*, London: Macmillan/Open University Press.

Wilkinson, R.G. (1996) *Unhealthy Societies*, London: Routledge. Wilkinson demonstrates that among the developed countries it is not the richest countries which have the best health but those with the smallest income differentials between the richest and the poorest.

Web sites

The healthy cities project web page (www.who.dk/healthy-cities/welcome.htm).

Department of Health (www.doh.gov.uk).

Chapter 6
Housing and urban development

Outline

This chapter will:

- outline the impact of urbanisation on the environment;
- describe the emergence of modern urban policy;
- consider the energy implications of housing;
- situate the discussion of sustainable housing in the context of contemporary urban policy.

Introduction

Housing has many environmental consequences: house building consumes raw materials and energy and the resulting development affects the wider environment. During the lifetime of a house a considerable amount of energy will be used in heating, lighting and all the everyday activities of life which require electricity. The location of households has implications for roads, schools, shops and other facilities. The decisions that government and local authorities make about the location of housing affect not only the lives of millions of people but also the landscape and the natural habitat. The present government policy is that 60 per cent of the housing required to accommodate the estimated 4.4 million extra households expected by 2016 should go on land previously used for another purpose and that is now vacant. These 'brownfield' sites are usually to be found in urban areas. Many people fear that unless this is done then a massive building programme on greenfield sites will erode the countryside significantly. The demand for more housing is a major national policy decision with nationwide implications in many areas where there is increasing conflict over the siting of developments. This chapter reviews how the present distribution of housing emerged and the environmental impacts of contemporary housing policy before considering the key elements of a sustainable housing policy.

Urbanisation

World-wide, urbanisation is proceeding at an alarming rate. Every 3 days, 1 million more people become city dwellers. In 1940, only London and New York had over 5 million people, but in the 1990s over twenty-two cities had more than 8 million inhabitants (Instituto del Tercer Mundo, 1997: 40). Globally, this process is consuming resources at an unprecedented rate, for all these millions of new city dwellers require water, energy and food. The demands they place on the rural hinterland are considerable, albeit significantly less than the demands those city dwellers in the affluent world place on the urban environment with their high-consumption, high-waste lifestyles. How the poor world responds to urbanisation is set to be one of the crunch questions for the future of humanity and the environment. If it mimics the hedonistic way of life of the affluent world, which is placing an insupportable burden on the planet, then there simply will not be enough clean water, energy or food to go round. Already, military strategists are talking about resource wars being among the coming armed conflicts of the twenty-first century. This involves those of us in the affluent countries as well, for we cannot expect the peoples of the poor world to moderate their aspirations and expectations while the affluent countries continue to party on with the world's natural resources.

Urbanisation in the UK

Cities pre-date industrialisation by several millennia. The urban form was bequeathed to Western Europe by the Greek city states and imposed on Europe by the Roman Empire. Medieval cities were often developments of a Roman plan. The industrial revolution changed this, for it created an urban area in what was once merely a village solely because it happened to be close to coal or water supply. Industrialisation, which started in the middle years of the eighteenth century, meant that factories and mills were hungry for labour; the migration of people to the industrial areas in the late eighteenth and early nineteenth centuries produced serious housing and health problems. The hectic building of houses to accommodate the new workers created overcrowding, sickness and disease. In these new urban settlements, the workers lived close by the factory, as did the factory owners. It took the best part of the nineteenth century before government recognised the dimensions of the urban housing problem. From the late nineteenth century, government gradually responded to the housing needs of the urban working class with legislation to clear slum areas and to allow for the construction of local authority housing. But it was not until after World War II that development and planning powers were given to local authorities which enabled them to respond to the housing and social need in a comprehensive manner.

Transport

Transportation created the urban shape. In the early years of industrialisation, this was foot power, so that workers had to live within walking distance of their job. The arrival of railways in the 1840s enabled people to live further from their place of work, although it was only the more prosperous who were initially able to take advantage of this form of mobility. The introduction of 'workmen's fares' in the late nineteenth century was to make this a real choice for many more people. The same process occurred with the car. At first, in the 1890s and 1900s, it was exclusively for the rich, then in the inter-war period its use was extended to the middle class, and finally in the 1950s the age of mass motoring arrived. The process of suburbanisation – the building of residential areas which related to the centre of the city – had begun with the railway, and the train and the car created many more suburbs in the twentieth century. To move out of the city into a suburb became a rite of passage for many people, signifying that they had reached a certain stage in their lives, which usually involved the arrival of children and the desire for a garden and proximity to green spaces in which to rear the next generation.

Suburbs

The suburbs were the first refuge for those who could not afford city life or who wanted some trees and open spaces in their lives. Since the decline of public transport in the post-war period, suburban living has put more strain on the environment. As car dependence grew, then the journeys became longer, and as bus usage declined so evening and unpopular services were deleted from the timetable. This, in its turn, increased pressure on people to become motorists. Out-of-town facilities have mushroomed until we have now reached the point where out-of-town shopping and out-of-town leisure developments are being joined by out-of-town employment as some firms relocate to the periphery or even to the countryside itself. In the USA, suburb to suburb commuting accounts for 40 per cent of journeys to work (Katz, 1994).

Garden cities

A century ago it was commonplace among social reformers to argue that the urban problems of overcrowding, poor sanitation, poverty and slum housing could be tackled by a variety of environmental solutions. Among these was slum clearance, which began in a small way before World War I. However, the garden city movement led by Ebenezer Howard quickly captured the imagination of a new generation of architects and urban reformers. In his book *Garden Cities of Tomorrow*, Howard (1902) outlined a solution to the key social problem of the day. Garden cities would take the excess (unemployed) urban population and provide them with jobs and good quality homes which had large gardens to be used as allotments to grow food. It took a while for the idea to gain financial backing, but the first garden city was begun at Letchworth in 1905 and this was joined by Welwyn Garden City in 1919 (Howard, 1902; Hall and Ward, 1998).

Garden cities were influential with architects and planners, and the garden city idea was taken up in a modified form by many of them. The suburban housing boom of the 1930s incorporated the green spaces and the tree-lined avenues espoused by Ebenezer Howard's design. The 'new towns' of the post-war years owed much to his work – among them Stevenage, Harlow, Basildon, Peterborough and Crawley.

Green belt

Since 1947, the Town and Country Planning Act has safeguarded rural areas from the sprawl of ribbon development and the pressure of housebuilding on greenfield sites. Green belt land has been designated in order to stop a process of sporadic but continual erosion of countryside for housebuilding. In large part, this has been successful, although it is open to local authorities to appeal to central government if they feel that there is a strong and compelling reason to build on greenfield sites. What it has not prevented is the post-war loss of population in cities.

Car dependence

The motor car has changed urban areas, small towns, the countryside – in other words, our lives – to an unprecedented extent. Cities throughout the world have attempted to adapt to the car, to give it more space on the roads, to allocate car-parking spaces, to build major highways and motorways and to demolish old communities to build new roads. In 1952, there were 2 million cars on Britain's roads, but by 1995 this had increased to 21.4 million (Potter, 1997: 2) and by 2001 had reached 23 million (Walters, 2001). The creation of out-of-town superstores and associated developments has led to greater use of the car. In the USA, employment and housing has been built alongside the retail parks to form a new urban environment – 'edge cities' (Garreau, 1992).

Urban policy

The retreat from the city began in earnest in the 1960s, when the mass ownership of the private car made it possible to commute not just from suburbs but also from country areas to city employment. Cities which owed their existence to the industrial revolution found that as these industries were unable to compete with wage rates and production in other countries then, inevitably, they closed. Industry, commerce, jobs and people have been leaving the city in large numbers over the last 25 years. This has been caused by industrial decline along with a mismatch of skills and jobs in the area – the new jobs do not require the skills that the local people possess. Social policies from the 1960s attempted to deal with the human effects of this in the USA and UK through community development and neighbourhood renewal (Higgins, 1978).

In the 1980s, these policies were augmented by economic regeneration schemes led by government quangos such as the Urban Development Corporations that were entrusted with important planning and investment powers – many of them taken from local authorities – and that were able to replan large areas and attract new investment. That the economic regeneration of old urban areas can occur is not in dispute, for example central Manchester or London's docklands, although the evidence elsewhere in the UK is more ambiguous. The population that is left behind in old urban areas is usually unskilled, often unemployed and marginal. The new jobs that are created in 'down town' areas usually require education, training and skills which the local population do not possess.

Over time, as more people moved out of cities, it became feasible for major employers to take advantage of the new roads infrastructure – the motorways and the expanded A roads network – in order to relocate places of work. This dispersed nature of post-war development made it less sustainable than previous housing and working patterns and is another result of the refashioning of the city and its hinterland to accommodate the car. The car has also encouraged longer journeys to work. Travel to and from work accounts for 19 per cent of all journeys over 1 mile, of which 75 per cent are made by car (Royal Commission on Environmental Pollution, 1997: para. 4.11). Those people living in smaller settlements tend to have the longest journeys to work (Potter, 1997: 19). The dispersal consequent upon car-based housing policies means that there are insufficient densities to sustain adequate bus services. In many suburban settlements, walking is inordinately time-consuming because of the low-density housing and it is not feasible to reach the shops on foot. Where houses are built forms one part of the sustainable housing issue – the impact of the houses once built on the natural and global environment is also extremely important.

The key reasons why cities have lost population are: (1) industrial decline with a mismatch of skills and jobs in urban areas and (2) slum clearance programmes which led to large, poor estates in inner-city areas and a constant move of people with job opportunities into the suburbs (Power and Mumford, 1999). The outmigration of middle-class and prosperous working-class people has meant that in some cities the inner-city schools have a high percentage of children who come from poor homes which are not motivated towards high achievement in education. Schools are a very important consideration in the location decisions made by parents when looking at housing as 'school performance affects neighbourhood prospects' (Power and Mumford, 1999: 37). City schools, particularly those in the central areas, have a reputation for poor results which discourages middle-class parents as they would prefer not to have to pay for private education if they live in the city. Inner-city areas are often a good location for single young people and couples without children and certain redevelopment schemes have targeted this group successfully.

Safety is another reason behind the loss of population and this is a particular concern for women. City streets can be frightening at night and those who can afford to do so often protect themselves by driving a car instead of using public transport or walking. Under local authority planning systems, many urban areas are zoned according to functions, i.e. chiefly residential, commercial or industrial. As a result, urban areas are often reserved solely for commercial and office use. They become empty at night because their sole population – the office and shop workers – have departed. Sometimes, the only other residents are the homeless, who sleep in the doorways and foyers of shops. In the Islington Crime Surveys of the late 1980s, 73 per cent of women and 27 per cent of men felt worried about going out alone after dark (see Worpole, 1992: 52).

These reactions are rational and cannot be discounted; the problems they highlight have to be addressed otherwise there is little chance that people will want to stay in the city if they have a chance to leave.

Country life

The British are one of the most urbanised peoples in Europe – 89 per cent live in urban areas – but sometimes it seems as though inside every urban dweller's soul there is an urge to migrate to the 'green and pleasant land' that he or she imagines the country to be. Just as the rich have passed down their aspirations for the good life of consumerism to the rest of us so their movement to the countryside, which began in the late nineteenth century, has in the twentieth century been copied by large numbers of 'those who are more modestly placed', as the Conservative government's Rural White Paper put it (Department of the Environment, 1995: 62). This migration became a significant factor in the post-war period. Large urban areas have seen a large-scale population loss, whereas at the other and of the spectrum there has been an increase in the population of small towns (Figure 6.1).

Many rural areas are now growing faster than urban ones. Between 1971 and 1996 the population of rural England increased by 24 per cent compared with 6 per cent across England as a whole. The days when agriculture was the major employer are long gone; nowadays, 73 per cent of jobs in rural Britain are in services, compared with 60 per cent in 1981 (Shucksmith, 2000).

One problem with this population movement is that an urban lifestyle in the countryside is maintained by continuing to work in the town or by driving further to the city. This has been referred to as the 'rurbanisation' process. The new residents, being car dependent, probably will not use the village shop (if there is one), preferring to travel to the superstore. Much of their housing is new build and this is preferred by developers, who can make greater profits on this kind of development. Developers make more money from the value of the land on greenfield sites, which is more highly sought after than brownfield sites. The market works against brownfield development in other areas as location is a very

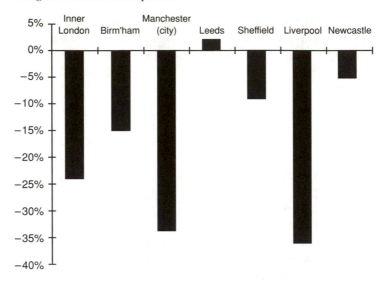

Figure 6.1   Population change in the urban areas of England 1961–94. Source: Office for National Statistics, *Regional Trends* (1997).

important factor in house purchase, and usually it is the case that inner urban areas are not highly prized by prospective buyers so higher prices cannot be charged (Rudlin and Falk, 1999: 113). Once established, new-build estates then generate demands for schools and other amenities and infrastructure, the cost of which has, in the main, to be borne by the local authority.

Rural inequality

Rural inequality is better disguised than urban inequality but is no less real for that. The movement of urban dwellers into the countryside has meant that house prices have risen out of the reach of many agricultural workers and those who have lived in the countryside for generations. Social housing might be expected to provide accommodation, but there is much less of this than in urban areas (only 12 per cent according to the White paper) (Reference). Second homes are sought after by wealthy town and city dwellers, with a consequent rise in house prices often putting them out of reach of local people. A 'gentrification' process is occurring in rural Britain as wealthier people outbid those on more modest incomes for scarce housing.

The countryside is not a place in which to live if you are poor. To obtain a job you almost always need a car, and many rural families will keep a car running in order to hold onto employment even though they cannot really afford it, thus reducing their spending on other items. This is a good example of transport inequality, for these are people who in urban areas would be able to use public transport. As the White Paper put it, 'private transport is now the key to maintaining the rural quality of life' (p. 74). Those who do not have access to a car then face social exclusion even more than those non-car drivers in urban areas. The number of bus kilometres operated in rural areas was cut by 25 per cent between 1950 and 1990, while the number of passengers fell by 75 per cent; 22 per cent of the rural population have no cars, 33 per cent are on low income or means tested benefits and 40 per cent are retired, unemployed or unoccupied (Boardman, 1998: 15).

The twin problems of transport and housing costs bear particularly hard upon young people, who find that in many rural areas a car is essential to get to work but the cost of running the car pre-empts money which could be used for other purposes such as renting property. Often, the solution is found by these youngsters staying in the parental home – with a consequent drain on the family's resources – and accepting that their wish to become independent will need to be delayed or it might mean leaving the area in order to find work in an area with lower housing costs (Rugg and Jones, 1999).

Where will we live?

Government projections in 1995 revealed that there would be an increase of 4.4 million households between 1991 and 2016 – an increase of 23 per cent (Rudlin, 1998: 3). This is produced by the rising divorce rate, the rise in the elderly population and the preference that many of us have to live as single-person households. Where to put the new households is an extremely sensitive – and potentially politically explosive – issue for it affects so many interests: builders, town planners, those resident in the countryside, those wishing to move to the country. The Labour government has announced that its target is that 60 per cent of the new housing should be built on brownfield sites – land previously used for building – although it enters the proviso that this is an overall figure which will be reached in some parts of the country, not reached in others and exceeded in some others.

The house-building industry believes that this is an unrealistic target and calls for greenfield building to be allowed, whereas Friends of the Earth advocates that 75 per cent of the new building should be on brownfield sites utilising a range of solutions – including housing above shops in city centres, building on land previously occupied by car-parks, increasing population density – which are part of the sustainable city agenda we will examine later in the chapter (Rudlin, 1998).

Urban renaissance?

What kinds of households will be created to compose the 4.4 million figure? Because of demographic changes, they will include a great majority of single-person households, although the married couples in this figure will be more likely to be childless than those in the past. Once these households have emerged, for whatever reason, what will they require in housing? The 'urban venturers' in their twenties will clearly want single-person accommodation. But many people are guided by what is available on the market. Since World War II, private developers have concentrated on building the 'family home', either detached or semi-detached. One of the problems with this ubiquitous design is that it consumes a lot of land and is resource intensive. Private developers prefer to build this type of housing on greenfield sites rather than on brownfield sites. Rudlin and Falk (1999) state the case for changing the priorities of builders so that they build much more single-person accommodation, arguing that this will need to be built on brownfield sites in order to reduce the pressure in the countryside. There are a number of locations which could be utilised for this kind of additional housing: car-parks, backlands – infilling disused land – utilising property over shops. But this raises the inevitable question of 'Will people want to live in urban areas?' It has been shown in major UK cities that there is a demand for inner-city living. But this comes primarily from young people under 30 without children. Whether the urban areas will attract older people and those in mid-life, with or without children, is less clear. Those people with aspirations for a better life – working class as well as middle class – generally conceive of this in a suburban or village setting but not in the city.

In 1998, the government appointed an Urban Task Force under the chairmanship of the architect Lord Richard Rogers with a brief to identify the causes of urban decline and recommend ways in which people could be attracted back into cities and towns. The report *Towards an Urban Renaissance* (Urban Task Force, 1999) outlines a range of fiscal measures which would induce city dwellers to remain in the city and make it more attractive for the suburbanites, such as council tax rates being slashed, VAT being removed to encourage renovation of property and stamp duty on house sales being removed. Rogers believes that it is still possible to turn urban decay into convivial cities with safe public spaces where pedestrians and cyclists are given priority and public transport is of a high quality (Urban Task Force, 1999). Some of this thinking was embodied in the Labour government's White Paper on urban policy which was published in the autumn of 2000. This announced tax incentives designed to encourage investment in urban areas, new planning guidance to encourage more people to live in urban areas and more measures aimed at creating employment in inner-city areas (Department of the Environment, Transport and the Regions, 2000).

Employment and housing

One of the most telling arguments against the urban renaissance school of thought is that it is out of line with employment trends. During the last two decades, there has been a deconcentration of jobs from urban areas to small towns and the countryside. Over 15 years starting from 1981, conurbations lost 0.5 million jobs, while small towns and rural areas gained 1.5 million jobs. It is the suburbs, small towns and rural areas which are fast becoming the new centres for jobs. Britain's twenty largest cities lost 500,000 jobs in the last two decades of the twentieth century, while the rest of the country gained 1.7 million (Breheny, 1999; Turok, 1999).

A significant factor influencing choice of housing location is employment. This is more complex than it used to be because of dual careers in modern families; usually, two journeys to work have to be considered. From the USA comes evidence that employees like greenfield sites for their place of employment just as much as housing (Garreau, 1992), and the new information and knowledge-based industries can be based anywhere – they do not need the city in the way that older businesses relied on its infrastructure. If this is the case then the old attraction of the city fades – for it will not be close to the place of work.

In thinking about the future shape of the city and the countryside, the environment in its broadest sense has to be considered. The problems of global warming and ozone depletion mean that carbon emissions have to be cut drastically. The Inter Governmental Panel on Climate Change estimated in its 1990 report that a reduction in carbon dioxide emissions of at least 60 per cent was required to achieve stability in the world's climate. This would mean that on a per capita basis the UK would need to implement a reduction of 90 per cent in carbon emissions. The Labour government is committed to keeping carbon dioxide emissions at 1990 levels until 2010. It means that there has to be a presumption against the out-of-town development which has been the hallmark of property developers over the last two decades and definite measures to reduce domestic energy consumption in addition to cutting back on car use. These are the dimensions of the problem of sustainable housing which faces government in the early twenty-first century. The problem can be simply stated: how can we best minimise the environmental impact of the new households we can expect to form in the next two decades while maintaining access to employment and the other amenities which are a necessary component of modern life? Before considering the policy options, we need to consider the environmental impact that houses make.

Energy

The housing of people living in traditional, preindustrial societies make much less of a demand on the environment because they use local materials, utilise natural energy as much as possible and, of course, do not have in-house electricity, water, central heating, air-conditioning or any of the other comforts which form part of the industrial, urban culture. In the industrialised West, these services are estimated to account for around 50 per cent of total energy use (Vale and Vale in Blowers, 1993). If transport – much of which is generated by the location decisions of home owners – is added, then the figure becomes 80 per cent (Owens in Breheny, 1992: 80).

The contribution to energy use made by housing is revealed in the following European Commission figures: energy consumption in European cities is composed of residential sectors and tertiary sectors, i.e. health, education, recreational services, and together these account for 40 per cent of total energy use whereas industry and transport account for 30 per cent each (European Commission, 1996: 114).

It has been calculated that the 'typical two storey dwelling house, with road space and drains, uses 80 tons of aggregate (including 12 cubic metres of concrete), 10 cubic metres of fired clay, 9 cubic metres of kiln dried wood, 12 square metres of glass, and significant quantities of more energy intensive materials' (Fairlie, 1996: 62). The consumer preference for the semi-detached or detached property has been bad news for the environment as they use more energy than the traditional terraced properties. Private house developers favour semi-detached and detached houses, asserting that they are popular with the public and therefore do not see any need to change their building style.

It is easy to forget how relatively recent the provision of indoor energy has been; after all, it was only in the 1880s that domestic water supply became a reality for working-class people in this country and it took another 50 years before gas and electricity became standard in most homes. To switch on a light or the central heating are such routine acts that we tend to forget the immense technological effort that goes into the production of the required energy. It is only at times of crisis that this is highlighted, as when the miners' strikes in the 1970s and 1980s led to serious shutdowns of domestic energy supplies.

Since the privatisation of the energy utilities – British Gas in 1986 and the electricity companies in 1990 – energy companies have reduced the price of energy on the domestic market. Electricity prices have fallen by 15 per cent in real terms while gas prices have been reduced by 16 per cent (Department of the Environment, Transport and the Regions, 1999b: 31). Although good news for consumers, clearly this is detrimental to long-term environmental policy because cheap energy contributes, through the emission of carbon dioxide, to global warming and is counter to the UK government's commitment to reducing carbon emissions.

UK governments have retreated from the positions they adopted at the time of the oil crisis in 1973. Then, the government, seriously worried by the large increase in the price of oil by the oil-producing states, introduced a policy of nationwide energy conservation. Grants were provided to insulate lofts and for draughtproofing and other energy conservation measures. These have survived into the 1990s as the Home Energy Efficiency Scheme but are now restricted to low-income households. Under this scheme, grants are given to those on low incomes or disability benefits, and people aged 60 years plus get a grant of 25 per cent of the cost of the work. The scheme can provide help with roof insulation, cavity wall insulation and draught proofing.

Although this ensures that the financial assistance is directed to those households where – without financial assistance – the work would not be carried out, it does mean that much energy conservation is left undone in other more affluent households because the grant is not there as an inducement. A scheme which was available to all households would benefit consumers, who would have lower energy bills, and the power generation industry, which would have less need to invest in new power stations. Overall, energy conservation has not received the attention it deserves, for it could result in a substantial saving in energy output. Under the Home Energy Conservation Act 1995, each local authority is required to produce a report on energy conservation in its area outlining measures which could be taken to improve energy efficiency.

Fuel poverty

The government definition of fuel poverty is the condition where households need to spend more than 10 per cent of income in order to keep warm (Department of the Environment, Transport and the Regions, 1999b). There are varying estimates as to how many households this includes, but it is in the range 5–8 million households; the wide range is caused by the differing definitions of income in the statement above, i.e. whether it is gross income or disposable income. Each year in the winter in the UK, 30,000 more people die than would be expected given the average death rate (Figure 6.2). The majority of these are over 60 (Department of the Environment, Transport and the Regions, 1999b: 8).

Measures to discourage profligate use of energy can conflict with policies to help the poor, simply because fuel is a much more expensive item for them than other income groups as they spend a

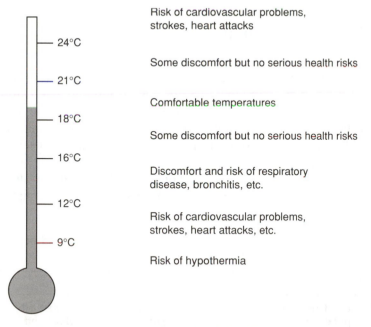

Figure 6.2   Room temperature and associated risks. Source: Department of the Environment, Transport, and the Regions (1999b: 8).

larger proportion of their income on fuel. In addition, those living in fuel poverty tend to have homes which are not well insulated. Many people living in social housing have expensive electric central heating systems which cost less than other systems to install, thereby saving the local authority money (Boardman in Bhatti *et al.*, 1994). Investment in insulation and cheaper forms of heating systems would help not only to reduce the bills of the poorest households but also to reduce their use of fuel. As Table 6.1 demonstrates, energy conservation is the best option for low-income consumers and the environment.

The domestic sector accounts for 30 per cent of the UK's total energy consumption and can be expected to increase as the number of households grows. The entire amount of electricity consumed by appliances has increased by 93 per cent compared with 1970 (Consumers' Association, 1999). These figures need to be set against the government's pledge to reduce greenhouse gas emissions.

Water consumption

All the water used in our homes is of drinking water quality, yet it does not need to be. For all our domestic household water needs, we use on average 140 litres daily, which is more than a bathful. 'Grey' – recycled – water could be used. For example, the water that has undergone the complete cycle in the washing machine could go through a domestic recycling facility and be used for flushing the toilet.

A properly sustainable house would recycle and reuse water in this way. Unless this is done, the demands of water consumption

Table 6.1 The effect of policy initiatives on the fuel poor and environmental pollution

Initiative	Homes	Planet
Increased income	Warmer	Worse off
Fuel price rise	Cooler	Better off
Investment in energy efficiency	Warmer	Better off

Source: Bhatti *et al.* (1994: 112).

from the projected 4.4 million extra households may well not be met by the water companies. The greatest demand for new housing is in the south-east of England, a region which has a water shortage problem because of the heavy demands placed upon water supply. The south-east is earmarked to take a substantial percentage of the new houses that will be needed for 2015, and if this building goes ahead on greenfield sites then there is a risk to water supply not only from the increased number of users but also because the underground springs which supply much of the water in this region will not be able to cope with the demand.

Sustainable cities

Why is it that today many greens emphasise the importance of city life and advocate a 'sustainable city'? They do so because for all their imperfections, environmental and economic, cities are still a less environmentally damaging way to organise the administration of business, finance, commerce, housing and employment than sprawling suburbs or out-of-town urban areas which encourage greater car use and energy consumption. High concentrations of people can live in cities and can be combined with a good public transport system and the promotion of walking and cycling. Mass transit systems efficiently transfer large numbers of people from their homes to the centres of cities. For all their imperfections, cities remain the most benign form of human settlement that is compatible with a way of life which expects domestic water, heat and power. But rurbanisation, edge cities and ever longer journeys to work amount to a future which will be even more detrimental to the environment. The proponents of sustainable cities argue that there have to be strict controls on out-of-town developments, greater toleration of mixed land use along with a much increased programme of energy conservation, restrictions on the use of the car and a major investment in public transport (Elkin *et al.*, 1991; Sherlock, 1991).

Herbert Girardet (1999: 13) believes that 'a sustainable city is organised so as to enable all its citizens to meet their own needs and to enhance their well-being without damaging the natural world or endangering the living conditions of other people, now or in the future'. This is an ecological aspiration but it is arguably the kind of vision needed if we are to begin to reverse the environmental damage which current urban settlements produce. It is worth bearing in mind that Ebenezer Howard's ideas of the 'garden city' were, a century ago, regarded as utopian. A sustainable vision of the city is imperative because the city is becoming the place where most people live. In 1900, only 15 per cent of the world's population lived in urban areas, whereas today more than 50 per cent live in urban areas, with the expectation that this will rise to 60 per cent by 2025 (Girardet, 1996b). The vast majority of people in the affluent world expect to enjoy the infrastructure of an urban existence, and in the poor world these expectations are increasing although the reality for many urban dwellers is a life of unremitting poverty in a shanty town on the outskirts of the city. This is not to deny that to live in low-impact developments, built of wood and local products, without these services is far less damaging to the environment (Fairlie, 1996). Major cities in the rich world consume vast quantities of goods from all around the globe, while the mega-cities in the developing world are sucking rural labour into their urban areas at an unprecedented rate.

'A city with a million inhabitants on average consumes 625,000 tonnes of water, 2,000 tonnes of foodstuffs, and 9,500 tonnes of fuel daily. It produces 500,000 tonnes of effluents, 2,000 tonnes of solid waste, and 950 tonnes of air pollution' (Sachs *et al.*, 1998: 150). Cities in the rich world consume materials and goods from all over the globe.

The ecological footprint is the total amount of energy, food and resources required to sustain an urban area. In the case of London, its footprint amounts to 125 times its present land area.

A sustainable – or compact – city organised in accordance with the principles of sustainable urban development would be a city where there was high-density housing, priority given to walking and cycling as transport modes with discrimination against cars and active promotion of public transport. Traffic calming in all residential areas would ensure that streets were liveable places where children could play freely and there was a good deal of social interaction. Zoning would not operate and there would be mixed use of areas with offices, shops and residential accommodation side by side.

These ideas were given some authoritative backing by the European Commission report on compact cities. It argued for a 'high density' mixed-use city where growth is encouraged within the boundaries of existing urban areas, but with no development beyond its periphery (European Commission, 1996). Most of the ideas surfaced again in the Urban Task Force report in 1999.

Conclusion

The question of urban regeneration is urgent if the inner-city areas are not to be locked into a spiral of decline with poor housing, poor schools and a declining population. The challenge is to attract new building into the centres of cities, often on brownfield sites, so that cities remain centres where people want to live and to work. This island is too small to allow some of the dispersed employment and housing which has become so popular in the USA. But, apart from this, there remains the crucial question of the transport infrastructure which will need to have a low-energy, more localised form based around public transport, cycling and walking. The impact of buildings on the environment is multifaceted as they consume energy, use materials and consume water. In all these areas, there are now well-tried technologies which reduce the impact of housing on the environment.

Key points

- Cities in the UK have lost population while small towns and suburbs have grown in size.
- Energy requirements of housing are a significant contributor to global warming.
- Transport has enabled people to live at greater distances from their place of work, but the increase in the length of journeys to work has adverse environmental consequences.
- For all their imperfections, cities remain an efficient way of providing services for large numbers of people.

> • How much new building occurs in urban areas and how much on greenfield sites is the key question for sustainable housing.

Guide to further reading

Girardet, H. (1996) *The Gaia Atlas of Cities: new directions for sustainable urban living*, London: Gaia Books. Attractive guide to a multitude of sustainable urban ideas.

Huby, M. (1998) *Social Policy and the Environment*, Buckingham: Open University Press.

Satterthwaite, D. (1999) *Sustainable Cities: an Earthscan Reader*, London: Earthscan. Brings together a wide range of material covering health, environmental justice, transport, industry and sustainability indicators.

Smith, M., Whitelegg, J. and Williams, N. (1998) *Greening the Built Environment*, London: Earthscan.

Urban Task Force (1999) *Towards an Urban Renaissance*, London: E and FN Spon.

Web sites

Council for the Protection of Rural England (www.cpre.org.uk).

Countryside Agency (www.countryside.gov.uk).

Department of Transport, Local Government and Regions. There are pages which contain the urban policy documents discussed in this chapter (www.urban.dltr.gov.uk).

Joseph Rowntree Foundation (www.jrf.org.uk).

Town and Country Planning Association (founded by Ebenezer Howard) (www.tcpa.org.uk).

Chapter 7
Food

Outline

This chapter will:

- situate UK food production in the global context;
- outline the developments in food retailing and relate these to social change;
- discuss the relationship between food poverty, poor diet and the diet of children;
- describe the food risks to health;
- examine the policy responses of government.

Introduction

Wherever we live food is basic to our survival; large parts of the world contain millions of people who live on a subsistence income with barely enough food. The impact of natural disasters and climatic change has obvious and alarming consequences for many of those living in the poor world because the accumulating evidence on the likely impact of climate change suggests that food supplies are in danger. Rising sea levels and changed weather patterns threaten to knock out some of the major grain-producing regions of the world. In those countries where there is no system of state income support, the rural poor who live in these areas depend on what they can grow from the land. Landless labourers in the developing world are increasingly attracted by the promise of a better life in the rapidly growing urban centres and they further intensify the urban demand for food. Food policy in the UK has to be seen in this global context: what we eat is often produced thousands of miles away and the decisions about what gets onto the shelves of supermarkets are influenced by international agreements and the multinational food corporations. Health, poverty and food have become inextricably linked. The discussion of food policy is inherently about health and so the risks to our health from consumption of certain foods is both a health and an environmental issue. There are various roles for the state in food policy: it can intervene directly by denying some people food choices or by rationing food, it can provide food to certain groups in the population, for example free milk or vitamins for children under 5 years old, and it can issue vouchers which can be used to purchase food (Leat in Murcott, 1998). In this chapter, we examine the nature of the debate about food policy and address its global dimensions.

The global context

While in the rich, industrialised world there is food in abundance and the highly processed, sugar-laden diet is prejudicial to the health of the population in the poor world, food shortages threaten human health and life itself. An impoverished and inadequate diet means that people are less able to fight disease. The average calorie intake in Western industrialised countries is in excess of 3,500 per day, but it is less than two-thirds of this amount in sub-Saharan Africa and South Asia (Conway, 1997: 1).

The processed, meat-rich diet of the affluent countries is responsible for damage to the ecosphere. Many forests have been lost to beef production. The cattle needed to produce the meat-rich diet popular in the wealthy world are themselves major consumers of grain which could be eaten by the world's poor. It takes 7 lb of grain to produce 1 lb of beef and 4 lb of grain to produce 1 lb of pork (*Independent on Sunday,* 10 November 1996). Grain stocks are at an all time low. Apart from the 80 million new people added to the world's population each year, the growing affluence of many people world-wide means that they consume more grain. As people become more affluent then they choose to eat more meat, e.g. the

Chinese are developing a taste for pork, poultry, beef, eggs and milk with the result that China is importing much more grain in order to feed animals. World grain stocks have also been depleted by the succession of climatic changes – heat waves, droughts and heavy rainfall have all damaged agricultural output.

The global food system is predicated upon high energy use, but only around 10 per cent of this is used in production, the rest being used for distribution and marketing (Tansey and Worsley, 1995: 223). Food miles – the distance travelled from farm to plate – have grown enormously because of the global system which aims to satisfy the tastes of Western shoppers all year round while producing environmental costs in the shape of pollution and fossil fuel use.

The Common Agricultural Policy (CAP) has been a major factor in UK agriculture and food policy since the UK joined the European Community in 1972. It has been the key influence on the way in which farming is conducted in EU member states. Established to support food production and the livelihoods of farmers, the CAP operates via a system of subsidies and intervention in the market, which means buying up surplus food in order to keep the prices higher than would otherwise be the case in a free market. The CAP was established in order to increase production and the system of price support for farmers meant that consumers paid more than the world price for food. Although they have been reduced, the subsidies are still considerable: in 1997, agriculture in the EU received a subsidy equivalent to 42 per cent of the value of its production compared with the subsidy received by US farmers of 16 per cent (Barnes and Barnes, 1999: 299). In this system, the rewards go to the bigger farms, which has meant amalgamation of small farms and the spread of intensive farming methods. There are now calls for the CAP to be used to achieve environmental objectives. These include increasing the amount of agricultural land which is devoted to organic crops, which represent a mere 2 per cent of agricultural land in the UK (House of Commons, 2001).

Modern farming

How we eat, what we eat, how we cultivate and how we use the land for agricultural purposes goes to the heart of the environmental question. Indeed, it is still the case that for many people the environment is the countryside – a powerful symbolic force in the nation's consciousness. This countryside has become an agricultural estate which produces food in abundance: the primary activity is the cultivation of crops for food and the rearing of cattle for food. The fact that it is able to do so is a direct result of the twentieth century invention of chemical fertilisers which have enabled large tracts of land, not previously farmed, to be brought into cultivation and the crop yields on existing land to be substantially increased. This has brought substantial dangers in its wake. Indeed, Rachel Carson's (1962) book *Silent Spring* exposed the dangers to human health from pesticides and lead, and the banning of DDT (dichloro-diphenyl-trichloro-ethane) was the real beginning of the contemporary environmental movement. At that time, it was recognised that, although DDT killed insects, the residues of DDT entered the food chain, leading to the production of thin-shelled eggs in some birds, which produced a decline in their numbers. Today, pesticides have an indirect effect by depopulating the countryside of its bird life for they kill off the food that birds eat, such as the weeds, insects, slugs and snails. The look and sound of the countryside has been changed by mass production techniques as hedgerows have disappeared and there has been a marked decline in bird numbers: familiar species such as skylarks, song thrushes and the grey partridge have all declined greatly in number while some rarer species have all but vanished. The Royal Society for the Protection of Birds concluded in 1996 that 'Farming that becomes so efficient, squeaky-clean with weed-free landscapes, ultimately leads to a bird free countryside, empty of wildflowers, butterflies, grasshoppers and birdsong' (RSPB, 1996, in Huby, 1998: 47). Meadows which are home for wildlife have disappeared because of the pressure of intensive dairy farming and cereal production (Wilson, 1999).

Food retailing

The ability to purchase good quality and reasonably priced food depends upon access to food outlets. These have declined substantially over the last three decades. There has been a major reduction in the number of local, small, corner shops which is directly related to the growth of supermarkets, first in city centres and High Streets and, since the early 1980s, in out-of-town locations. So much so that today the big four – ASDA/Wal-Mart, Sainsbury's, Safeway and Tesco – control 85 per cent of the UK food market. The dangers of monopoly power and the restriction of choice are well known, but for social policy the problem is more that this monopoly reduces food choices for those who are disadvantaged. There are now 'food deserts', i.e. areas where there are no food shops for local people, necessitating a journey to shops at some distance made that much more difficult if one has to use public transport.

The major players in the food industry have a stranglehold on the market. They have achieved this at the expense of smaller competitors and closed many traditional small retailers – not only food shops but also pharmacists, newsagents and florists. In a small way, new alternatives are now emerging which aim to supply the perceived deficiencies of the food business in this country. Organic food (see Box 7.1) co-operatives supply to their members organic food at a cheaper rate than that to be found in shops.

Although operating on a small scale, farmers' markets are another way of getting fresh fruit and vegetables to people, and much of this is organically produced. The markets – which originated in the USA over two decades ago – are organised so that local produce can be sold straight from the farm. They help to

---

Box 7.1 **Organic food**

Produced without the use of artificial fertilisers and pesticides. Crops and animals produce the natural balance. Crop rotation is used to keep soil fertile and not chemicals. Animals are not routinely given medicine.

reduce the problem of food miles bearing in mind that in the USA the average carrot travels 2,000 miles before it is sold whereas a farmers' market carrot travels an average of 50 miles (Festing, 1998a: 41).

Eating habits and cooking

There has been a considerable change in eating habits since 1945. During the first 10 years after the end of World War II, government played a major role in the distribution of food via the system of rationing introduced during the war, which was not finally dismantled until 1954. Shortly after the end of the war, the National Food Survey was started in order to monitor what it was that people were eating. This survey of eating habits has continued since then. Currently, it monitors the expenditure patterns of households. Rationing was designed to secure an equitable distribution of food, and, as well as this, it did have the effect of reducing the social class gradients in the consumption of nutrients. After the end of rationing in 1954, there was a big surge in demand for food which had been difficult to obtain, such as meat, eggs and canned fruit. Sugar consumption rose rapidly in the post-war period, so that by 1960 Britain had the fifth highest consumption per capita in the world. Refrigerators in homes were another extremely important development in the 1950s, for these and the later appearance of home freezers and microwave ovens provided the technology for the dramatic increase in the use of convenience foods.

Convenience food took off in this country with the precooked meal, which needs little preparation other than microwaving or boiling in a bag. The sales of these ready meals have rocketed in the last two decades and are related to the entry of women – the traditional meal-makers – on a large scale into the workforce. The UK now has the largest market for ready meals in Europe. Another firm favourite with the British public is ready-to-cook pizza; again, this would appear to be because of its convenience as in the first half of the 1990s consumer expenditure on pizza rose by 55 per cent. Because of their convenience, pasta and rice have now become staple parts of the UK diet (Mintel, 1997).

Knowledge about the preparation of food has declined to the point where it is possible to say that the UK population has become deskilled in the sphere of cooking. The shift to a much more technological approach to cookery – now renamed food technology in the National Curriculum – is but one example of this. There is a remarkable process going on within education, with old skills such as cookery and domestic science being phased out while there is an increasing emphasis on teamwork, communication and information technology skills. Greens would argue that deskilling is part of the package of contemporary Western societies with their excessive emphasis on material consumption, and Greens would want to promote cooking as it is part of self-reliance.

It is clear that there is little point in exhorting the population to eat a more healthy diet if many people do not have the skills to cook nutritious meals. In the case of those people who eat their main meal in front of the television, one would assume that they did not want to invest time in cooking a meal when they could use convenience food. As Fieldhouse (in Lang *et al.*, 1999: 3) has commented, 'if prepared food is so easily accessible, why bother to learn to cook? If you haven't acquired cooking skills, then fast foods are the most efficient answer'. Community food schemes which teach food preparation skills obviously have a place but they are aimed at people living in low-income areas, whereas the evidence from recent research suggests that the lack of cooking skills is to be found across social classes. Initiatives to support the sale of fresh fruit and vegetables in inner-city areas and outer estates with no shops are important. The government has recognised the significance of access to shops selling basic goods and fresh fruit and vegetables by sponsoring shops doing just this in areas which have been abandoned by retailers and are now 'food deserts'. The cultivation of fruit and vegetables is important in a national policy for food and there is concern about the loss of allotments.

Between 1970 and 1996 there was a massive decline in the number of allotments, with almost 10,000 allotment plots per year being lost (Stott, 1998). There are real fears that a commitment to building on brownfield sites will mean the loss of even more allotments at a time when government is stressing the importance of physical exercise and eating fresh fruit and vegetables.

Food poverty

The social investigations of Booth and Rowntree which exposed the nature and extent of poverty 100 hundred years ago were, in part, about access to food and the way in which poor nutrition appeared to be the norm for large sections of the working class. There was growing concern from the beginning of the twentieth century about the consequences for our armed forces if the underfed babies and children of the time should grow into men who were unfit to serve in the armed forces. There were two main responses to the revelations on the extent of underfeeding and poor diet. Many argued that the income of working people needed to be increased to enable them to purchase enough food of the right quality, while there was another view that working-class families had enough income but they spent it on the wrong things, e.g. money which should have been spent on food was spent at the betting shop or the public house. Philanthropists devoted a considerable amount of time to instructing working-class women on the importance of budgeting and thrift, although this was a part of the working-class culture which had also created friendly societies and thrift clubs. Social reformers who believed in higher wages for working people might also subscribe to the view that more education was needed about the importance of a balanced diet and budgeting. In the inter-war years, the nutritionist Sir John Boyd Orr exposed the deficiencies of many people's diets in poor areas with the publication of *Food, Health and Income* in which he claimed that 'a tenth of the population, including a fifth of all children, were chronically ill-nourished, while a half of the population suffered from sort of deficiency' (Stevenson, 1984: 215). World War II led to increased wages and a reduction in unemployment which produced an improvement in diet. By the 1960s, Royston Lambert observed that the evidence of the National Food Survey demonstrated that 'Family size and composition are now the principal determinants of nutritional status in our society. Small or childless families have made substantial nutritional gains in the decade but the diet of families with three or four children or with adolescents and children has shown no overall improvement and some notable falls in nutritional adequacy absolutely and relatively since 1950' (Lambert, 1964: 45).

Today's literature on food poverty shows the lower intake of nutrients among the poorest in our society. Men and women in manual occupations have a poorer quality diet than those in non-manual occupations. When money is short, it is often food which is cut back in order to pay for other items. Typically, in families, parents will reduce their food consumption in order that there is more food available for the children. There are real difficulties in obtaining fresh fruit and vegetables now in many low-income areas because of the movement of food retailers into out-of-town retail centres (Killeen in Fyfe, 1994). One inner-city resident remarked of their area 'It's easier to buy drugs than fresh fruit and vegetables – and there is more selection' (Leather, 1996: 32). Smoking compounds the vitamin deficiency problem. Smokers have lower concentrations of iron and vitamin C and the pattern of smoking corresponds to a social class gradient, with the poorest having the highest level of cigarette consumption.

The lack of a car often prevents a shopper from accessing the lower prices to be found in out-of-town superstores. Car-less shoppers are usually reliant on the dearer, local shops unless they can get to the city centre, although the major food retailers have closed many of these stores in favour of out-of-town locations (Raven *et al.*, 1995). In the UK, food expenditure is proportionately much higher for poor families than for those on middle incomes. Those in the lowest decile of income spent 25 per cent of their incomes on food compared with 14 per cent in the highest decile (Central Statistical Office, 1995).

Poor diet

Although there are those who experience food poverty, for most people in the UK there is an abundance of food available. Yet the food we eat has become, for the most part, too processed, too high in sugar and too manufactured, with the result that obesity is a growing problem together with weight-related diseases. In 1976, the Department of Health identified coronary heart disease as a major health problem in its publication *Prevention and Health: Everybody's Business* (Department of Health, 1976). Diet was among the factors in the cause of coronary heart disease alongside lack of exercise and smoking. Doctors now recommend a diet with lower levels of sugar, salt and fat and an increase in the intake of dietary fibre. The advocates of a healthy diet have had some success in their efforts to get Britons to adopt better ways, e.g. the sales of skimmed milk has increased and the numbers of vegetarians has risen. Our diet, though, has to be seen as part of our way of life, and unfortunately some social trends encourage unhealthy eating. The emergence of dual-earner households where time is at a premium has meant that there is less time for cooking and meal preparation – indeed, less time spent in the eating of the meal. Convenience food has become a major part of the British diet. Dinner is often a pizza eaten in front of the television rather than a meal prepared by a family member in the kitchen and eaten at the dining table. The introduction of interactive television means that it is now possible to order a take-away pizza without leaving your armchair. The 1993 Health Education Authority Health and Lifestyles Survey found that one-third of the people sampled reported that they ate their main meal in the living room in front of the television (Lang *et al.*, 1999: 31). Microwave dinners are designed for this kind of meal. As a nation, we are eating out more: on average, families spent 20 per cent of their total food expenditure on eating out in 1990 compared with 10 per cent in 1960 (Cooper, 1995b). It is estimated that 30 per cent of disposable income in Britain is spent on eating out (O'Hara, 2000), and the British consumption of chocolate has increased over the last two decades, making us third in the world confectionery consumption table (Harding, 1997). The results of these changes in eating behaviour are seen in the increased number of overweight people. In the UK between 1980 and 1992, the overweight and obese rose to 54 per cent of men and 45 per cent of women (Hunt, 1996). The figures for obesity have worsened in the 1990s: 16 per cent of women were obese in 1993 compared with 20 per cent in 1998, whereas 13 per cent of men were obese in 1993 but 5 years later it was 17 per cent (Boseley, 1999). The implications of these trends for body weight, body shape and fitness levels are serious. This is especially true for children.

Children's diet

Children consume a diet in which fatty foods are conspicuous. The National Diet and Nutrition Survey, published in 1995, showed that under-fives had a diet high in sugary and fizzy drinks, white bread, savoury snacks, chips and confectionery and low in leafy green vegetables, raw vegetables and salads (Department of Health, 1995). A comparison of the diet of 4-year-olds in 1950 with that of 4-year-olds in the 1990s revealed that despite rationing and austerity the 1950 children had healthier diets. They had higher calcium and iron intakes and consumed less sugar. Table 7.1 shows the very low consumption of soft drinks and sweets compared with children in the 1990s. Children of all ages consume unhealthy food – snacks, crisps, sweets – in such large amounts because of the

Table 7.1 Children's food consumption, 1950 and 1993, showing average daily grams of food groups consumed by children aged 4 years

	1950	*1993*
Pasta, rice, etc,	<1	31
Bread	120	48
Biscuits	4	17
Milk puddings	71	9
Milk	307	247
Yogurts	0	23
Eggs	32	9
Spreading fats	20	7
Meat (beef, lamb, etc.)	24	21
Poultry	<1	11
Fish and fish products	7	10
Leafy vegetables	13	6
Root vegetables	3	11
Other vegetables	54	35
Potatoes	75	66
Fruit and nuts	36	51
Preserves, spreads	15	2
Confectionery	<1	25
Tea	194	35
Soft drinks and juices	13	446

Source: Meikle (1999).

enormous advertising expenditure of food manufacturers aimed at children. A report in 1995 by the National Food Alliance found that children watched three to four times more advertising for fatty and sugary foods than adults. Seventy per cent of advertisements shown during children's programmes were for food compared with only 20 per cent during adult programmes (Cooper, 1995a). The phenomenon of 'snacking' among children has contributed to the poor diet of the nation's youngsters.

School meals used to provide one nutritionally balanced meal among a daily diet of crisps, lemonade and chocolate, but there has been much disquiet about the nutritional status of school meals since 1980 when the government removed the nutritional standards stipulation. The National Heart Forum claimed that too many secondary schools were providing school meals that were high in fat and sugar. School meals had to be supplied by private firms from 1988 under the Conservative government's compulsory competitive tendering initiative, and it is alleged that this resulted in caterers using more prepared food and sugary snacks in order to cut costs. 'National Heart Forum statistics revealed that 46 per cent of calories in school meals studied came from fat compared with the government's recommendation of 35 per cent. They found that each week the average teenager consumed four packets of crisps, six cans of fizzy drinks, seven chocolate bars, three bags of chips and seven puddings while only eating one seventh of the recommended intake of fruit and vegetables' (Cooper, 1995a). Given this diet of the average teenager, it is important that the school meal is properly nutritionally balanced, but this is only part of the solution for so many school children's midday meal – the packed lunch – is determined by their parents and consists of crisps, chocolate biscuits and white bread sandwiches, a diet which will exacerbate any tendency to excess weight.

Overweight children present a challenge for the future health services. Children do not get the exercise that they used to enjoy in the past from playing on the streets, far fewer walk to school and they do not for the most part use their bikes as a form of transport. This reduction in physical activity has meant that there is an increased tendency to weight gain and many children have high blood cholesterol levels. Inactive children have a tendency to become inactive adults, with the attendant problems of overweight people and increased risk of coronary heart disease, adult-onset diabetes, hypertension, obesity, osteoarthritis and osteoporosis.

Food and the environment

The UK food retailing industry is part of a global market which ensures that strawberries are available for UK shoppers all year round (at a price!) and exotic vegetables are there whatever the season. This incurs enormous energy costs in moving food vast distances to satisfy the palate of the Western consumer. 'Food miles' refers to the distance travelled from the farm to the plate, and with some items this can now be measured in thousands of miles. The costs to the environment include pollution, road maintenance and fossil fuel use.

Food packaging is another environmental problem. All those containers and packets need to be disposed of either in incinerators or in landfill sites. A US estimate was that about 12 per cent of solid waste came from food packaging (Sennaur *et al.*, 1991: 289). In the UK, each family buys £10 worth of packaging each week (Lang and Hines, 1993: 94). It has been calculated that only 10 per cent of the fossil fuel energy used in the world's food system is utilised in the production of food – the remaining 90 per cent goes on distribution and marketing (Tansey and Worsley, 1995).

Food risks

Nowadays, the most common media stories about food are to do with food scares: the risks of illness, or even death, resulting from certain foods or food products. Public alarm has been fuelled by growing evidence that it is possible for disease in animals to be transmitted to humans. The discovery of bovine spongiform encephalopathy (BSE) or 'mad cow disease' in cattle that resulted from sheep remains being put into the feed for cattle was extremely damaging for the UK meat industry, with a mass cull resulting in the loss of 8 million cows and a ban on exports of British beef to the rest of the world. Most alarming was evidence that it can be transmitted to humans through cheap beef products, such as beef burgers, in the form of CJD (Creutzfeldt–Jakob disease). Seventy people had died from CJD by 2000 in Britain, with the incidence growing at 20–30 per cent a year. Public concern has been heightened by the evidence that carriers of variant CJD who are incubating the condition may not display any of the symptoms but are able to infect others through contaminated instruments in hospitals or dental surgeries (Meikle, 2000).

Food risks have sadly become commonplace (see Table 7.2). In 1988, the then junior Health Minister, Edwina Currie MP, was sacked when she remarked that most of British egg production was infected with *Salmonella*. Subsequently, the annual number of deaths attributed to *Salmonella* has fallen: in 1990, there were around seventy deaths, but in the late 1990s there were around thirty deaths per year, although there has been a yearly increase in *Salmonella* poisoning from 10,000 to 30,000 during 1982–96. *Escherichia coli* (*E. coli*) 0157, a bacterium found in raw and undercooked meat, has claimed scores of lives during the 1990s. There has also been a rise in *E. coli* 0157 poisoning from zero to 600,000, and a rise in *Campylobacter* poisoning from 25,000 to 45,000 (Meikle, 1998).

Genetically modified food

Whether or not there are risks to human health from the consumption of genetically modified (GM) food is now hotly debated. The GM food debate (Table 7.3) has revealed the extent of the public unease about food production. Genetically modified foods are being sponsored by major companies, principally in the USA, which see them as extremely important in increasing crop yields. Using gene technology, it is now possible to transfer different characteristics among plants, e.g. some plants have been made resistant to weedkillers by this process and some produce their own insecticide. Supporters say that genetic modification has the capacity to increase yields and to increase the flavour and the shelf-life of foods. One of the most attractive arguments put forward for this new food technology has come from Gordon Conway, who argues in his book *The Doubly Green Revolution* (Conway, 1997) that GM food offers the developing world a way to feed a growing

Table 7.2 Food poisoning

	Description	Symptoms	Where it gathers	Transmission
Salmonella	A rod-shaped bacterium	Diarrhoea, vomiting, abdominal cramps, fever	In the gastrointestinal tract of wild and domestic animals, birds, reptiles and occasionally humans	From red and white meats, raw eggs, milk and dairy products, yeast, sauces, chocolates, cream-filled deserts
E. coli 0157	A bacterium	A serious inflammation of the colon which leads to blood in the urine and can be fatal	In the gastrointestinal tract of healthy cattle and possibly domestic animals	Beef and beef products and unpasteurised milk, raw vegetables, yogurt, cheese, meat pies; can be spread person to person by direct contact and by direct contact with animals
Campylobacter	A group of spiral-shaped bacteria	Abdominal pain, profuse diarrhoea, nausea, vomiting	In the gastrointestinal tract of birds and animals, cattle and domestic pets	Raw or undercooked meat (especially poultry), unpasteurised milk, domestic pets with diarrhoea

Source: Meikle (1998).

Table 7.3 Genetically modified food

For	Against
Health benefits as GM food can be better balanced for nutrition, e.g. crops could be grown which had more amino acids, reduced levels of fat	Risk; we do not know the potential risks which will result
GM food could help to end world hunger as it would be possible to store food longer and produce more nourishing crops	Power concentrated in the hands of large agri-business
GM food can be produced which does not spoil so readily or is tastier or cheaper	The technology is uncertain; gene transfers can lead to unpredictable outcomes
Fewer pesticides and herbicides needed	Putting toxins into plants to engender resistance could create superpests; new allergies and toxins have been reported

population and in so doing to improve its chances of economic and social development. Working with the United Nations' definition of 'food security' – 'access by all people at all times to enough food for an active, healthy life' (Conway, 1997: 287) – Conway argues that the science of genetic manipulation should be put to work for the benefit of the poor countries through increasing yields and producing disease-resistant crops. Yet one has to be cautious about this line of argument for the track record of multinational companies' involvement with poor countries in agriculture is not a good one as many countries have moved into a position of monoculture – producing one crop for the world market – and yet not seen their economy prosper as a result.

Food policy

During World War II, with the country in danger of being starved into submission by the Germans, food policy became of paramount importance for the effective waging of the war. The Ministry of Food was created to run the extensive bureaucracy needed to ensure that rationing functioned smoothly. Rationing did not finally disappear until 1954, when the Ministry of Food was merged with the Ministry of Agriculture. In reality, the merger of the two ministries was a take-over by the Ministry of Agriculture with food policy being marginalised. The interests of farmers were paramount and over-rode other considerations (Franklin in Henson and Gregory, 1993). During these post-war years, the official policy was to increase food production as much as possible, hence the official endorsement of factory farming and large-scale crop production. The price of food was to decrease significantly. At the European level, the CAP has been a major factor in British agriculture and food policy. The Ministry, which has been severely criticised for its bias towards farmers, has nonetheless had the responsibility for ensuring food safety, along with other arms of central and local government.

Post-war governments interpreted the consumer protection role of the Ministry of Agriculture as ensuring that health regulations or legislation affecting farming and food retailing were observed. The BSE crisis has starkly revealed the imperfections in the consumer protection system. The Ministry of Agriculture has long seen its role primarily as the body which works closely with the food producers and the farming interest, and this relationship is strengthened by an elaborate system of subsidies and grants and support schemes. This stance has incurred a barrage of criticism in this era of food scares. Critics have argued that a much more interventionist role is required of government, and this extends to government viewing environmental considerations as an integral part of food and agriculture policy. The creation of the Department of the Environment, Food and Rural Affairs may achieve this.

There are inherent conflicts in food policy among the food retailers, the public, the representatives of that public, i.e. the consumer organisations, the agricultural interest, the food-processing industries and the public and the environmental health departments. All have a stake in food policy, and government has the role of holding the link between these interests and protecting the consumer (Lang, 1997). The CAP of the EU is central to this process and has been a key influence on the way in which farming is conducted in EU member states. Established to support food production and the livelihoods of farmers, it operates via a system of subsidies and intervention in the market, which means buying up surplus food in order to keep the prices higher than they would be in a free market. In this system, the rewards go to the bigger farms, which has meant amalgamation of small farms and the spread of intensive farming methods. There are now calls for the CAP to be used to achieve environmental objectives, including an increase in the amount of agricultural land devoted to organic crops. Clearly, another environmental objective would be to increase the amount of food which is grown in the UK at the present time in order to reduce the food deficit, i.e. the big gap between the amount of food which is produced in this country and the amount which has to be imported.

Food Standards Agency

As a result of the BSE crisis there were many calls for a tougher government regime which would protect the consumer – many felt that a government agency which would have food safety as its number one mission was sorely needed. Shortly after being elected in 1997, the Labour government announced that a Food Standards Agency (see Box 7.2) would be created which would monitor the food chain 'from the farm to the shop or restaurant' (Ministry of Agriculture, 1998). The role of the Agency has been carved out of

---

Box 7.2 The role of the Food Standards Agency

- Monitor the safety and standards of all food for human consumption
- Advise on diet and nutrition
- Lead or share in the lead on investigations into food poisoning organisms, animal feed, food hygiene, genetically modified food and additives
- Co-ordinate and monitor law enforcement in food safety
- Commission scientific research

an existing division of responsibilities between the Department of Health, the Ministry of Agriculture and local authorities. The agency has monitoring, auditing and co-ordination tasks. Much of the food law enforcement remains with local authorities, but the Agency has the ability to ensure that they do carry out this work. It was also envisaged that the Agency would be able to take over unusually complex litigation.

In establishing the Agency, the government recognised that concerns over food safety were no longer the sole province of the Ministry of Agriculture. Inevitably, real questions remain as to the extent to which the Agency will be able to police the activities of major food suppliers, retailers and agri-business. Genetically modified food is one vivid illustration of a technology that will need to be closely monitored, but it is unclear to what extent the Food Standards Agency will be involved in the decisions regarding its future in the UK.

Conclusion

Nature provides the wherewithal for food production, but humankind's relationship with the land is in crisis. Our food makes us sick; its methods of cultivation and production ensure environmental problems for the poor world; the distance that some food has to travel is wasteful of energy.

The world population explosion presents a new challenge for global food policy. As we have seen, GM crops are one possible response, although a green agriculture sees GM as the latest in a line of environmentally damaging agri-business solutions which include pesticides and herbicides. Green agriculture puts a premium on local food production and organic methods, arguing that the farmers in Africa and other malnourished parts of the world would be better employed in the long run producing food for themselves and their communities rather than growing cash crops for export to the rich world. The risks to human health resulting from agricultural practices have demonstrated that a food policy is needed in this country. The Food Standards Agency is designed to ensure that food safety and the health of consumers are addressed. But access to healthy food and the knowledge needed for its preparation are also extremely important for the nation's diet and are important aspects of the social policy of food.

> **Key points**
>
> - UK food production is part of a global food system based upon high energy use.
> - The development of food retailing has reduced food choice, particularly for poor people.
> - Food risks have led to the establishment of the Food Standards Agency.
> - Food policy needs to ensure access to low-cost healthy food and to promote cookery.

Guide to further reading

Huby, M. (2000) 'Food and the environment', in May, M., Brunsden, E. and Page, R. (eds) *Social Problems in Social Policy*, Oxford: Blackwell. Situates food policy within the wider social and environmental context.

Murcott, A. (ed.) (1998) *The Nation's Diet: the Social Science of Food Choice*, Harlow: Longman. A collection of papers from the ESRC research programme on 'The Nation's Diet'.

Piachaud, D. and Webb, J. (1996) *The Price of Food: Missing Out on Mass Consumption*, London: London School of Economics. Reports on the impact of modern food retailing on disadvantaged people and reviews possible solutions.

Tansey, G. and Worsley, T. (1995) *The Food System: a Guide*, London: Earthscan. Sets out the global context of food policy.

Web sites

Department of the Environment, Food and Rural Affairs (DEFRA) (www.defra.gov.uk).

Food Commission (www.foodcomm.org.uk).

Food Standards Agency (www.foodstandards.gov.uk).

National Association of Farmers' Markets (www.farmersmarkets.net).

Chapter 8
Work

Outline

This chapter is about the ways in which alternatives to a consumer society are emerging and offering a different way of responding to the wants and needs of people. The nature and meaning of work in advanced industrial societies is explored with a review of employment in the UK, and the future of employment, the position of those excluded from employment and consumerism will be outlined. In the second part of the chapter, we will look at some alternatives to mainstream thinking. These include Citizen's Income Local Exchange Trading Systems and the redistribution of work.

We are fixated, both as a nation and as individuals, by the employment organisation. Work is defined as employment. Money is distributed through employment. Status and identity stem from employment. We therefore hang onto employment as long as we can; we measure our success in terms of it; we expect great things from it, for the country and for ourselves and we cannot conceive of a future without it.

(Handy, 1984: 188)

A century ago overwork was a sign of poverty. Today it is a sign of wealth and prestige.

(Mulgan, 1997: 93)

Introduction

Work has been pivotal to social policy in the UK for centuries. The Poor Law system was constructed around work. For the 'able bodied' (fit adults) to receive assistance from the Poor Law, there was the requirement to enter the workhouse. The modern social security system is designed to promote incentives to work symbolised in Beveridge's depiction of 'idleness' as one of the giants that had to be slain. Since its election in 1997, the New Labour government has introduced its 'welfare to work' policy designed to enable young people and single parents to enter work and leave the benefits system.

Employment – paid work – is a the centre of the process of industrialisation which is transforming our world. The agricultural workers who are leaving the rural villages in Africa, Latin America and Asia exchange a pattern of life in which work is a part of a centuries-old culture based around family and kinship for the paid employment of the city, where it is no more than a cash relationship symbolised by the contract. The raw material of the natural environment has been the means by which humankind using physical and mental labour has been able to create technologically based industrial societies. The industrial system depends on raw materials, minerals, the seas and rivers and the energy derived from mineral deposits. These modern societies are of a relatively recent origin in the annals of time: 250 years ago all human societies were based around agriculture and subject to the domination of nature. Now, we have got to the point where we are able to speak of the 'end of nature' (McKibben, 1990) as nature has been irredeemably altered by our actions. It remains to be seen whether humankind can construct ways of working which reduce the damage to the planet and yet enable the world's population to live a decent life. Work is central to our identity and human culture but the contemporary organisation of work is damaging for the environment, individuals and society.

Green utopians are clear that the industrial system puts an enormous burden on the planet which will result in an environmental crisis of gigantic proportions. Their solution is a drastic one: societies should deindustrialise. The relationship between the rich world and the poor world should be turned upside down, with rich countries aspiring to the simplicity of the way of life to be found in rural parts of the poor world. Whether such visions of deindustrialisation are appropriate or feasible is open to question, but it should be noted that a growing unease about the centrality of paid work and consumerism is now gradually emerging across the political spectrum.

Work enables us to participate in the consumer society, to afford the 'good life' as defined by the advertising industry. Because the modern world is predicated upon the idea of work as paid employment, we can forget that this is a particular way of looking at work which privileges that work for which payment is made and demotes the importance of unpaid work. Paid employment performs a number of functions apart from providing money – it offers many people the opportunity to feel valued and a part of their community, it sometimes provides human contact for many people who otherwise would feel isolated in their homes. In the consumer societies that have been created in the rich world, one of the functions of money is to provide a passport to enjoying the goods and services which we need for our daily existence. Money provides a status which enables participation in many activities in the society while consumer goods denote one's status to others – the Gucci or Rolex wristwatch will impress some people. But this economic system, although it has produced untold wealth, has its costs: the environmental resources that are required to sustain high-consumption societies are immense, while the pollution produced as a result of increasing energy is a major cause of the warming of the planet.

In our 'work and spend' society, those on low incomes or on benefits find it hard to feel that they are full members of that society. Millions in the UK are excluded by the fact of unemployment or disability or caring responsibilities which mean they cannot join the labour market. The human consequences of the way in which production and consumption are organised cannot be ignored, for in the affluent countries there is a significant group of the population that is not sharing in the benefits of the consumer society – a group that may well consist of unskilled workers living in a region of industrial decline or disabled people or school leavers without any qualifications. Nonetheless, by comparison with the standard of living of the majority of the world's population, they are rich, but understandably they compare their lot with the lifestyles of the affluent they see portrayed on the television every day.

Employment in the UK

Between 1960 and 1980, the UK was transformed from a manufacturing to a service economy. The loss of millions of industrial jobs had a big impact on the low-skilled and unskilled male workforce. Unskilled men are more likely to be unemployed than other workers and more likely to remain unemployed for longer.

By contrast, women's employment has risen sharply, although in part this is because of an increase in the number of part-time jobs which appeal to women, who often wish to combine paid employment with caring responsibilities (Hakim, 1996).

The twin pillars of the post-war period between the mid-1940s and the mid-1970s were the welfare state and full employment – a society where there was a job available for anyone seeking one. The collapse of full employment in the mid-1970s set off a train of rethinking about employment across the political spectrum. The transition to a service-led economy produced numerous social and economic changes and created numerous losers as well as winners. This was a shift from a society built around production – a full employment society which equated with full-time, lifelong employment mainly for men – to a consumer society where employment is no longer a lifelong job but more a series of jobs, and the labour market has been feminised to the point where approximately half the workforce is female. There has been a trend to flexibility of working practices in the UK economy over the past two decades, which has meant that part-time and contract employment has come to the fore; the majority of these posts are filled by women rather than by men, a fact which needs to be borne in mind when one compares the overall percentage of women in the workforce. Flexibility in labour markets has been supported by governments over the last two decades through privatisation and the opportunity extended to the private sector to tender for government services. Government has responded to the rise in unemployment by innumerable training schemes for the most vulnerable workers, seeking to equip them with the necessary skills and abilities to gain employment in the new labour market. As society has become more mobile with the rise of private transport, the geography of employment has changed. Cities and towns no longer have the Victorian employment map with the major employers in the centre with workers living on the outskirts or suburbs. Because the majority of workers have cars then often it will be the rural location to which firms relocate. That one-third of households where there is no access to a car find it most difficult to access employment.

The neglect of public work

At the same time as the big shift was occurring in the economy from the manufacturing to the service sector, local and central government was undergoing a transformation in the way it operated. The techniques of the private sector were imported into the public sector: efficiency, effectiveness and economy became the watchwords of the new public management. Services which previously had been supplied in-house were contracted out to firms who competed for the business. Local authorities were put under pressure to employ fewer staff. The net result was that a great number of tasks were no longer performed as they were too costly or it meant that too many staff would need to be employed. This has had a visible impact upon the social fabric: many parks were replanted with annual plants, thus saving the labour of tending plants from year to year; park keepers disappeared; railway stations were dirtier as the interval between cleaning lengthened; the number of station staff was reduced to save money; there was less street cleaning; and public spaces were neglected. Work was not being done in order that budgets could be cut.

It only requires a walk around the streets of an urban area to see how the reduction in the numbers of people employed in public services has led to a visible deterioration in the quality of urban spaces: more dog dirt, vandalised toilets and bus shelters, litter and pavement parking.

Time deprivation and commodification

There are some households that are 'work rich' – where both partners are earners and through their work contacts can obtain other part-time employment or contracts if they so desire – and some that are 'work poor' – where both partners are living on social security and are cut off from the networks which would alert them to job opportunities. Paid work has become the essential aid to accessing the consumer society, and it is reaching ever deeper into households. Children work, often illegally, from 11 or 12 years of age and it is not uncommon to find teenagers working while at school, not just 'Saturday jobs' but other days of the week as well. This carries on into higher education, with many university students working during term time

The time squeeze experienced by dual-earner households means that in many households the traditional tasks done by women – taking responsibility for the cleaning, cooking and overall management of the household – are done by domestic labourers of one description or another: nannies for the children, cleaners for the house and other services. Overwhelmingly, this work is performed by women and is low paid. The professional middle class now rely upon a domestic service economy composed of child-minders, nannies and cleaners. This has grown considerably in the last two decades, and it was in 1994 that it was reported that there were more nannies in the UK than there were car workers (Demos, 1994). Normally, the relationship between the cleaner and the professional middle-class woman is profoundly unequal – with the cleaner not having the same opportunities open to her. Some commentators predict that this kind of relationship will be seen much more in the future, with the lowest income groups getting employment by servicing the needs of the rich and the 'contented majority' of the middle class. They will be a service class providing personal services which their employers do not have time to perform themselves. The inequalities in earnings have increased as a result of the dual-earner professional middle-class family.

Time deprivation is now a recognised phenomenon, and the consumer society responds to this by commodifying many of the activities that previously were part of everyday family life. Companies provide the services which consumers do not have time to do themselves. Those who use domestic workers instead of doing the cleaning themselves and who get nannies to look after their children are commodifying this work. This is work which can be produced within the family, by parents and by other family members, but now many people use the market in order to get this work done for them. This in turn gives them more time to pursue their careers.

In the USA, there are innumerable firms which specialise in this work: Kids in Motion gets children from school to after-school activities; Beck and Call does errands of any kind; Playground Connections 'matches playmates to one another', in some cities; Precious Places helps parents decorate their children's rooms; Creative Memories puts family photos in albums (Hochschild, 1997). There are a great many other activities which have been commodified: household skills such as jam-making, sewing, knitting, bread-making. Very many people now lack these skills and have to use the market system in order to purchase them. There has been an extensive deskilling of the population for a great many reasons which are connected with the 'work and spend' society – it is too time-consuming, and it is too expensive to make things oneself because of the low cost of, say, clothes from poor world sweat shops.

The advanced societies are witnessing a celebration of wealth which makes the poverty of those on low incomes and state benefits the more difficult to bear. The Chief Executive Officers (Managing Directors) of America's largest companies earned thirty-five times as much as the average worker in 1973, but now it is over 200 times as much (Frank, 1999). The lifestyles of the rich trickle down for imitation to the rest of us. 'I've worked hard for it therefore I deserve it' is frequently used as a justification for purchase of yet another consumer durable. Globalisation is creating an international league of high-flyers who can command very high salaries because of their skills and knowledge.

Voluntary work

Our society's commitment to paid work leaves less time for other forms of work. The statistics show that there has been a decline in the amount of time spent on voluntary work in the UK, and the decline in voluntary work by young people is marked. The 1997 National Survey of Volunteering showed a sharp reduction in the levels of participation in volunteering among young people and found that young people had the most negative views about volunteering.

'If they have spare time they would rather work for money. They comment on the availability of part-time work and on the plethora of other outlets and diversions – and expenses – within youth cultures' (Gaskin, 1998). There may be many other reasons why young people may not want to volunteer – it is not regarded as cool or they would look a sucker among their mates if they worked for nothing. The lack of time for volunteering is seen most clearly in the USA, where the traditional voluntary organisations, the Girl Guides, the Scouts and St John's Ambulance Brigade have been hit particularly badly, just as in the UK. Women used to keep many of these organisations going, but now with the advent of the dual-earner family they are not available to take on these roles anymore. Men are not taking their place.

Time deprivation

Time is the good that the affluent lack. Time is spent and is organised – usually these days by a diary. The poor are rich in time but they lack the wherewithal to enjoy it in the way that a consumer society stipulates.

In this 'work and spend' society, money is the key to full participation. But this does not mean that money is used in order to purchase leisure, but rather money is used in order to free up more time for work. In both the USA and the UK, longer hours are being worked but at the same time much more is being spent on consumer durables and on domestic and other kinds of time-saving services. The health and social consequences of a long-hours culture are coming to be recognised on both sides of the Atlantic. In 1996, a survey of 1 million white-collar workers in the UK found that although three-quarters of them had contracts which specified that their working week was between 35 and 37 hours two-thirds of them regularly worked more than 40 hours per week and one-quarter more than 50 hours per week (Clement, 1996). Some sociologists have argued that because parents have less time for their children there is now a parenting deficit in the USA and the UK (Etzioni, 1995). Although it is a complex subject, it is not unreasonable to regard the strains produced in families by such long hours as a factor in the high divorce rate in this country.

The American writer Barbara Brandt refers to the 'job addiction' that pervades the USA, where one's worth and value come from having a full-time paid job. It is seen in the assumption held by some employers that the job is the most important thing that individuals do in their lives, more important than their marriage, their family or anything else (Brandt, 1995). This used to be called the 'male' organisation of working life with its cult of long hours – presenteeism – but it is now being aped by those women who have adopted the long-hours culture and the 'male' approach to work (Wilkinson and Howard, 1997).

The harm done to our lives is spelt out by Frank (1999: 5):

> All of us – rich and poor alike, but especially the rich – are spending more time at the office and taking shorter vacations; we are spending less time with our family and friends; and we have less time for sleep, exercise, travel, reading and other activities that maintain body and soul.

Having sketched the nature of the meaning of work in our society and the inequalities and diswelfares which result from this in a general way, it now remains to examine those alternatives which have come from green writers and others.

In the second part of the chapter, we can examine some green responses to the organisation of work in a consumer society, a society which is characterised by high rates of unemployment in certain areas and, for many of those in work, by time deprivation and a long-hours culture with a divide between the work-rich households and the workless households. The schemes that are outlined here are all providing work in what is now called the 'social economy' jobs created to meet needs which cannot be supplied by public sector services. Usually, this work is precarious, funded by short-term contracts and often from a variety of funders.

In the social economy, there is a mix of paid – if insecure – employment and volunteering. The needs which this sector supplies are vast and range from community care to environmental projects to provision for children.

Financial exclusion

Low-income areas, by definition, are short of cash. What little money there was would in the past have remained in the area because there were many more local shops and small businesses. Out-of-town superstores have effectively killed off the small shops and, most recently, banks have joined the migration from these areas.

One-third of bank branches have closed in the period since 1987 (Mayo *et al.*, 1998). Those branches which are first on the list to be closed are those that do the least business, usually to be found in low-income areas. It is not just individuals who suffer from this closure of banks, but the small businesses who operate in disadvantaged areas feel it acutely. They find it more difficult – just because of their small size – to get adequate start-up finance from the High Street banks.

The banks are investing heavily in internet banking. Internet banking is skewed heavily towards the south-east of England, users are more likely to be men, under 35 years and in the AB and C1 social classification (Treanor, 1999). But the banking system is becoming more remote for many people – the arrival of telephone banking and internet banking and the replacement of thousands of branches and staff by computerisation has meant that reasonable sources of finance are difficult to obtain.

In these circumstances, it is very tempting for residents to take advantage of the credit companies who specialise in loans to people who have a poor credit rating and thus would not qualify for a bank loan from a High Street bank. But these will often be charging exorbitant rates of interest, e.g. a £100 loan over 6 months where the repayment is £140 is equivalent to an APR of 250 per cent. The problem is that this credit is very expensive for the customer. 'Between 6 and 9 per cent of individuals lack either a current or a savings account; 75 per cent of people without accounts are unemployed or economically inactive, and 25 per cent of households in the UK, and over 50 per cent of the lowest income households, have no home contents insurance' (Mayo *et al.*, 1998: 6). The people without bank accounts are more likely to be women, young people, older people, unemployed people and the people on low incomes and living in rented housing (Pratt *et al.* in Conaty and Mayo, 1997). This financial exclusion debars the poorest from enjoying some of the benefits which credit can obtain for most people in our society.

Credit unions

Credit unions are a response to the financial exclusion which is to be found in many disadvantaged areas. They are co-operative organisations for saving and borrowing where members have to give a certain amount of money in order to become a member – a bond – which is then at some point re-lent to the members. There are about 175,000 members of credit unions in the UK. This is a small figure compared with the USA and the Republic of Ireland. Some of the bigger credit unions provide services such as home contents insurance, usually acting as an agent for an insurance company, as a catalogue company agent, for debt consolidation and rescue loans, specific savings and budgeting accounts, for example for Christmas, holidays, etc., and finally for bill payment (Conaty and Mayo, 1997: 8). The importance of credit unions is that they represent a secure and reliable source of funds for the poorest in our society, whose only other alternative would be the 'loan sharks' who charge exorbitant rates of interest.

Citizen's income

A citizen's income – which is also known as the basic income – would be a benefit paid as of right – no means tests or other criteria for eligibility – to everyone in the country who holds citizenship. Citizen's income is designed to support all those people who, for one reason or another, are not part of the mainstream economy, either because they cannot get a job or because they choose to work at tasks which are not part of the cash economy. No country has yet introduced such a scheme, but it is an idea which has come from the fringes of the social security debate to the mainstream. It would be paid regardless of the fact that one was a millionaire or an unemployed person with no other income. Citizen's income would also be paid without reference to one's previous work record – unlike the national insurance scheme where benefits paid depend upon contributions made in the past. It would be paid to individuals and not to families or households, without taking into account income from other sources. Supporters argue that this universal, non-selective approach is one of the particular strengths of the citizen's income, for it will end means testing. In that sense, it will be a recognition of the informal work that is carried out on each day without any monetary recognition, e.g. by those who undertake domestic labour (chiefly women) which at present does not even get included in the national accounts, although if a woman employs another woman to do her cleaning and pays her a wage which goes through the taxation system that is counted as part of the gross domestic product. Carlson (1997) concludes that citizen's income is by itself not going to achieve a change in the distribution of domestic work and caring tasks which at present falls mainly on women, although it might encourage more men to take part-time work and assume more domestic responsibilities. However, the factor which seems to produce an increase in men's contribution to domestic labour is women's full-time participation in the labour market.

There are variations on the citizen's income, e.g. Atkinson (1996) argues for a participation income because he does not think that a citizen's income is going to be acceptable to the country if it allows people to draw income without working in any way. For someone to be eligible for the participation income then they would have to do voluntary work or some form of community service (see the discussion in Fitzpatrick, 1999: 115–22).

The citizen's income is designed to help part-time workers and support job sharing. The green writer James Robertson makes a case for the citizen's income as a measure that will encourage self-reliance whereby people will be able to provide some services for themselves which at present they buy. The cushion of the citizen's income will enable voluntary work to revive, and there will be more time for caring. Robertson believes that people need to become more self-reliant – and hence withdraw some of the demand for waste-producing services – and the citizen's income would help to achieve this. He sees the citizen's income as returning to people their share of taxation, which increasingly will be eco-taxes, but believes that they must make further provision on top of this by using their skills and resources (if they have them). In so doing, they will be taking back for themselves some of the power over their lives they have ceded to others and living by their own resources and work (Robertson, 1996, 1998). Proponents of the citizen's income believe that it could replace all other social security benefits. It is an attractive proposal because it is socially inclusive, no one is excluded and there is no requirement to behave in a certain way in order to obtain the benefit. For greens such as James Robertson this is but one part of a broader strategy including a reform of taxation which would remove taxes from employment and place them firmly onto environmental pollution.

Citizen's income is a radical break with centuries of income maintenance policy in the UK because it severs the link between work and benefits – a link which has recently been reinforced by the government's 'welfare to work' policy. It is doubtful whether there would be public support for a citizen's income which would make payments to individuals regardless of their willingness to work. For many people, it would be seen as rewarding those who choose to be idle. For this reason, variants of a 'participation income' seem much more acceptable to policy-makers and public opinion.

A full citizen's income would necessitate an increase in the standard rate of tax, which makes it a non-starter for governments committed to low taxation regimes, unless, of course, the basis of taxation is changed and income tax becomes less of a yardstick by which the electorate judges governments.

Local exchange trading systems

Local exchange trading systems (LETS) are a form of barter, or agreement, between two people that they will pay each other an agreed number of tokens for a particular task. LETS have spread rapidly in the UK. In fact, there are more LETS in the UK than anywhere else in Europe. The idea was first put into practice by Michael Linton in British Columbia, Canada, in 1982 because he was disturbed at the way that wealth was leaving the local community (Dauncey, 1988).

In a LETS the usual procedure is for one of the members to act as the banker and keep a note of all the transactions that have taken place. With the widespread availability of personal computers this is much easier to do than it was in the past. All members of the group have the right to see the list of members and the tokens they have. The scheme members decide at the outset how many tokens will be awarded to each member and from then on it is up to each participant in a transaction to decide how many tokens they will pay the other for their service. Another initial task for those establishing a scheme is to decide how much the tokens will be worth in relation to the national currency. There is no compulsion for members to use the scheme once they have joined. A lot of the work done in LETS is the provision of services: domestic cleaning, car cleaning, cooking. Some people use LETS in order to learn a skill – a language, car maintenance, music, cooking – while some people hire goods which they do not possess, such as computers or lawnmowers. Naturally, it can be a problem if one member provides a lot of services and does not buy any in return, for if they carry on doing this and no new tokens are issued then it can lead to the scheme slowing down for want of currency. But they do not gain interest on their tokens as in a bank so there is less incentive to hoard them.

LETS have a directory of members and their services. Tokens are usually given names – the first LETS in the UK was at Stroud, so not unnaturally the tokens there were called Strouds. In Manchester, they are Bobbins; in Lewes, Trugs; in Southampton, Solents; in Newbury, New Berries; in Malvern, Beacons; in Totness, Acorns; while in Brighton, it is Brights; in Brixton, Bricks; and Canterbury has Tales.

This is one of the most important bonuses of a LETS – that it ensures the 'payment' stays within the area. This should be important in an area where most of the population live on low incomes or state benefits for, there, the little cash that is in circulation will often find its way into the tills of the major supermarket groups and out of the area.

Unfortunately, the experience in the UK has been that LETS are not booming in areas of high unemployment. It had been thought that they would be a good way to harness the unused skills and capabilities of people who are outside the conventional employment sector as they do not have a paid job. LETS would be a way in which people in low-income areas could begin to use the skills and services available locally, plugging people into a network of goods and services from which they are normally excluded by the cash economy. This has not happened to the extent that was envisaged. Instead, LETS have flourished in middle-class areas, often being strongest where there is an 'alternative' culture. In 1994, the New Economics Foundation surveyed the then 350 schemes and found only seven in low-income areas. In a recent review of LETS (see Table 8.1) operating in poor areas, Hudson *et al.* (1999:

Table 8.1 Potential of LETS to re-engage individuals into the local economy

Social exclusion can mean	*LETS offers*
Lack of money/income to buy materials needed to exchange in formal or informal production	Reduced need for money for buying goods or services which individuals may otherwise not be able to afford
Social isolation resulting in fewer chances to hear of work or other opportunities	A social network within which exchanges can take place
Lack of requisite skills or reduced chance to use existing or develop new skills	Skills development through exchange
Low self-esteem and self-confidence	Improved confidence for those not in paid work and greater sense of self-worth
High cost or difficulty accessing credit	Zero-interest credit
Low money circulation	High local currency circulation and trading

Source: Hudson *et al.* (1999: 9).

3) highlight the following barriers to its success: too few community activists who could 'champion' the idea; insufficient attention to marketing the scheme in language that local people can relate to; a lack of confidence among local people as to their skills and abilities; a limited supply of services on offer in the LETS ; a fear among local people that they could go into debt in a scheme; a fear of letting unknown people into the house – this was particularly felt by women.

The biggest obstacle to LETS growth in low-income areas may be the fact that the social security position has been unclear, and this might be a deterrent to would-be members and to the creation of new schemes. There does not seem to be any consistent approach by the Department of Social Security to LETS – in other words, the Department leaves interpretation to local officers and some have said that if someone is active in a scheme then they are presumed to be unavailable for work and therefore should not receive benefit. However, the fact that work for LETS can be done at any time does mean that this is a somewhat strange interpretation of the rules. Another real disincentive for social security claimants is that their benefit might be reduced pound for pound if the local office deems that their LETS work is equivalent to cash. This is beyond the earnings disregard of £5 or £15 per week depending on whether they are unemployed or lone parent claimants. Another possible way in which their benefit could be affected is if it is deemed that they have worked more than 16 hours in a week. However, it would be most unusual for anyone to spend this amount of time on LETS work. People claiming to be sick could be refused benefit on the grounds that if they are in a LETS then they are not unfit for work (Barnes *et al.*, 1996). At present, the government is considering the option of allowing claimants to keep up to the equivalent of £1,000 before their benefit is affected.

The idea behind linking the LETS to the national currency is that it makes it easier for businesses to join. If a business is a member then obviously this makes the scheme more attractive to some people who can then use its services where previously they would not have been able to because of the lack of cash, and, at the same time, it makes the scheme better known. In some areas, the local LETS currency will be taken as full or part payment in cafés or at the local farmers' market. It is the self-employed business person who is most likely to get involved with a LETS . There is a real problem for a business if it cannot in the course of its work use the credits it has accumulated and this would considerably reduce the attractiveness of a LETS to the business.

There are now many examples of LETS being supported by local authorities as part of their commitment to sustainable development. They supply development workers in some areas and can help LETS get in touch with other organisations who might be interested in working with them. Or a LETS can be used to support a group of people who find it difficult to obtain work in the conventional economy, e.g. people with mental health problems.

LETS could well play a significant part in a strategy to provide services and help for people outside the mainstream economy, but they clearly need financial and administrative support in order to grow.

Time dollars

Another way of harnessing the talents and time of people also comes from North America – the time dollars idea originated by Edgar Cahn. They are designed to meet the social needs which their founder feels are no longer met for a lot of people in modern society, such as companionship, love and caring. One time dollar is given for each hour spent on a task, but they are not in the main meant to be spent. Unlike LETS, a co-ordinator does the matching of volunteer to recipient of the service, and, like LETS, the records of work done are kept on a central computer. The scheme started in the early 1980s in Missouri, when people over 60 earned service credits by offering respite care. One advantage of time dollars is that they make volunteering more attractive to those who think that you are stupid not to receive money in respect of work performed for other people. Time dollars have proved themselves very useful in harnessing the labour of numerous volunteers in health care and personal social services. The largest system is in operation in Miami, Florida, where it is used for these services: 'housekeeping for the sick or elderly, deciphering Social Security rules, companionship, respite support for carers, lifts to the doctors, the church or the supermarket, letter writing, reading to the blind, pet care, baby sitting, language classes, sewing classes, and adult day care' (Douthwaite, 1996: 90).

Time dollars convert people's time which might otherwise be underutilised into an asset they can then use to purchase such services themselves when they need to. Time dollars are in their infancy in the UK, and still at the planning stage in a number of areas. What is clear is that they differ from LETS in that they are not a currency – they have to be used by the people who have earned them – they cannot be spent for services such as the local café would provide. Those elders in Missouri who read to the blind will be able, however, to use the time dollars they have earned to get someone to perform a service for them, such as mowing the grass. But only about 15 per cent of time dollars are actually spent in this way, so they are more akin to voluntary work (Boyle, 1999: 4).

Redistribution of work

Longer holidays, early retirement, job sharing and reduction of the working week to 35 hours are all proposals which would reduce working time (see Vail in Vail and Wheelock, 1998: 208–11). If there are work-rich and work-poor households then a simple solution might seem to consist in reducing the hours worked by those in full-time work and, hence, employers being able to employ more staff.

But, once stated, the objections are clear: would the workers who reduced their hours be paid the same weekly wage (in which case the employer would not be able to afford to employ more staff) and, if they are not to be paid their old wage but instead take a cut in their weekly wage, then why should they want to do this? A reduction in working hours is also recommended as a way to equalise the domestic burden of household labour, which at present is overwhelmingly carried by women. The reasoning is that men with more time on their hands will then devote it to household tasks, but of course this does not automatically follow. Clearly, this will be attractive to some workers, but others will surely wish to work longer hours and enjoy the consumer goods that they can then afford.

It would appear that the way forward for redistribution of work to occur is for the state to take a lead and finance schemes that will encourage the workforce to take non-waged work more seriously. Paid parental leave would be an obvious example where parents would be able to receive a wage while taking care of their small children in their early years. (The recently introduced UK government scheme does not provide for payment to parents.) An optimistic interpretation of the direction that the UK economy is taking would be that the growth in part-time jobs should enable those in marriages and partnerships to combine work and caring responsibilities.

Conclusion

Politicians know that people care about their jobs, savings and money more than anything else. A consumer society, because it fixates people on the goods that money can obtain, has a tendency to extinguish alternative ways of understanding. Money is a universal touchstone. In this chapter, we have seen how in the USA and in the UK over the past two decades the world of paid work has become so important and has sucked so many people into its embrace, including women and young people at school, while children suffer because of their parents' commitment to employment, which means that they see much less of them. For green thinkers, it is important to reduce the amount of time spent on alienating labour and increase time spent on 'own work', i.e. work which reflects a person's own interests. The schemes outlined here embody an alternative to the mainstream economy and provide opportunities for recognition of the vital unpaid work performed in society.

Unfortunately, there is little evidence to suggest that large numbers of people in consumer societies would want to end their commitment to the 'work and spend' society. Reductions in working time do not appear to be attractive, and one could envisage some workers having their working week reduced from 40 hours to 35 hours obtaining a second job to make up the hours!

The dynamic of this system is the ever more competitive global economy, which has meant that the UK has had to give up on much of its manufacturing industry because the goods can be produced much more cheaply in the poor world or China and the Far East. The market system now extends into areas of life previously undreamt of having vanquished its chief opponent – the Communist systems of the USSR and Eastern Europe. The next chapter outlines the implications of the new global system for the environment and social policy.

Key points

- Paid work is central to social policy and the income maintenance system has been constructed on this basis.
- The transition from a manufacturing economy to a service-led economy has produced a major increase in part-time employment and an increase in female participation in the labour market.
- Time deprivation means many household tasks are now becoming low-income occupations.
- Financial exclusion has led to an increase in credit unions.
- LETS and time dollars are useful means of ensuring that work gets done and services are provided in areas where employment is scarce.
- There is a role for the state in promoting schemes which enable employees to combine their caring responsibilities with paid work.

Guide to further reading

Boyle, D. (1999) *Funny Money: in Search of Alternative Cash*, London: HarperCollins. This is a readable account of local currencies based on the author's travels in the USA.

Douthwaite, R. (1996) *Short Circuit: Strengthening Local Economies for Security in an Unstable World*, Dartington: Green Books.

Fitzpatrick, T. (1999) *Freedom and Security: an Introduction to the Basic Income Debate*, London: Macmillan.

Vail, J., Wheelock, J. and Hill, M. (1999) *Insecure Times: Living with Insecurity in Contemporary Society*, London: Routledge.

Chapter 9
One world

Outline

This chapter considers the global context in which social and environmental policies are emerging. Globalisation and free markets have ensured new roles for multinational corporations and for non-governmental organisations. The complexity and scale of environmental and other world problems has led to calls for global governance. On the individual level ecological citizenship has been promoted as a philosophy which will be a suitable response to the environmental crisis, but can it flourish in consumer societies?

Introduction

Environmental problems are global problems: each week brings more news stories about the gathering environmental crisis across the world. Massive forest fires are fuelled by intense global warming, and the carbon from these fires makes global warming worse. Fish stocks are falling at an alarming rate. Species extinction continues apace. The melting of the ice at the Arctic is destroying the feeding grounds of the whales and walruses while polar bears and seals at the Arctic are in decline, and many parts of the UK have experienced severe flooding on an unprecedented scale. Most of these environmental problems have global causes. The overheating of the planet is the cumulative result of industrial processes in numerous countries. The holes in the ozone layer are the outcome of the accumulation of pollutants over many years across the world. When humanity disturbs the delicate and complex pattern of inter-relationships in the natural environment this has an impact in other parts of the world. Nowhere is this more clearly seen than with the pattern of global warming which is producing the movement of the currents, thus affecting the climate of many countries.

In this uncertain world, the last 10 years have been notable for the international co-operation displayed at conferences on the environment and sustainable development. The sustainability discourse popularised at Rio shows little sign of receding in international development and environment circles. There is a new global environmental context in which governments now have to operate, but at the same time they are confronted by a global economic order which has reduced the power of the nation state. This chapter outlines this global world order and then considers some of the implications for social policy.

Globalisation

Globalisation has a long history. It could be argued that the beginning of a global system of trade can be traced back to 1492 when Christopher Columbus presented himself at the court of the Spanish Queen Isabella and King Ferdinand and obtained the financial backing for his expedition which resulted in the discovery of the 'new world'. The Spanish Empire which emerged was rivalled by the British and Dutch and inaugurated an era of colonialism that opened up most of the world to the Western European powers and endured until the twentieth century. Is the present phase of globalisation merely a continuation of this process which has been in place for a couple of centuries? Proponents of globalisation argue for its novelty on two counts. The first is that the sophistication of modern communications technology means that distances have been considerably reduced, e.g. information can now flow round the globe in a matter of seconds while journeys which once took weeks are completed in hours. The explosive growth in communications technology means that it is now feasible, as distance times have been cut so dramatically, to move production from the rich world where workers have good welfare entitlements, wages and conditions of work to the poor world where labour costs are so much lower. So much manufacturing is now being done in China that it is fast becoming known as the workshop of the world.

As Box 9.1 shows, along with the new forms of communication technology there are also new actors in the shape of organisations and new markets.

The new means of world communication permit the global financial system to transmit trillions of dollars each day on foreign exchange markets. The size of these transactions is daunting, dwarfing anything else seen before. The rise of the multinational corporation is an associated phenomenon. These companies usually

---

Box 9.1 The global context

New markets

Growing global markets in services – banking, insurance and transport
New financial markets deregulated and working around the clock
Proliferation of mergers and acquisitions
Global consumer markets with global brands

New actors

Multinational corporations which integrate their production and marketing and dominate world production
The World Trade Organization – the first multilateral organisation with power to enforce national government compliance with rules
Growing network of international non-governmental organisations
Regional blocs – such as the EU – proliferating and gaining in power

New tools of communication

Internet
Cellular phones
Fax machines
Faster and cheaper transport
(based on United Nations Development Programme, 1999: 30)

have their headquarters in the USA or Western Europe, but have plants in many other countries. Multinational corporations are now among the richest institutions in the world, with some of them having larger GDPs than many countries (see Table 9.1). They are involved in more than 60 per cent of trade in the world today (United Nations Development Programme, 1999: 114): Globalisation means that multinational corporations are attracted to poor world economies because of their low labour costs which go hand in hand with poor social welfare. Corporations do not want to have to pay additional taxation in these countries in order to support social spending programmes. The reason why, after all, they have

Table 9.1 Top corporations and their sales compared with the gross domestic product (GDP) of selected countries in 1997

Country or corporation	GDP or total sales (US$ billions)
General Motors	164
Thailand	154
Norway	153
Ford Motor	147
Mitsui & Co.	145
Saudi Arabia	140
Mitsubishi	140
Poland	136
Itochu	136
South Africa	129
Royal Dutch Shell Group	128
Marubeni	124
Greece	123
Sumitomo	119
Exxon	117
Toyota Motor	109
Wal-Mart Stores	105
Malaysia	98
Israel	98
Colombia	96
Venezuela	87
Philippines	82

Source: United Nations Development Programme (1999: 32).

Note
Gross domestic product is the sum total of all money-based goods and services produced by the domestic economy in a year.

moved their factories to the poor world is that labour costs are cheaper, and part of the reason why this is so derives from the fact that they do not have to meet some of the costs of social provision.

Free markets

The second distinctive feature of contemporary globalisation is that it has a specific ideology of free markets. In this ideology, the market is the economic instrument which reveals the true preferences of the population through its choice of goods. Free markets are being introduced throughout the world because of the belief that this represents progress for humankind. Free market ideology has led to economic modernisation, i.e. the privatisation of state industries and the removal of barriers to foreign trade. It is assumed that this modernisation should take the same form in different countries, but there are serious grounds for doubting whether one model of a free market can fit every economy in the world and there is clear evidence that China and other South-East Asian economies are not going to accept the US model of the free market (Gray, 1998).

The agencies which promote this ideology of free markets are the World Trade Organization (WTO), the International Monetary Fund (IMF) and the World Bank, which all have their origins in the 1944 settlement reached at Bretton Woods, USA, when the World War II allied powers laid down the framework for post-war economic life. The World Trade Organization replaced the General Agreement on Tariffs and Trade (GATT) in 1995. It has expanded the role of the organisation from the regulation of international trade to include services such as banking, transport and telecommunications. It has the ability to impose trade sanctions on countries when it decides that they are not complying with WTO agreements. To date, this has meant that European and Japanese food safety measures have had to be withdrawn, as have US clean air measures and marine mammal conservation laws. The International Monetary Fund nowadays has a focus on assisting developing countries through its programmes of loans. It too is an enthusiastic advocate of free markets and ties its economic assistance to demands that social policy spending be cut along with the introduction of privatisation and removal of barriers to foreign trade. The World Bank – full title International Bank for Reconstruction and Development – makes loans to member nations at rates less than those of the commercial banks to assist with building the infrastructure of the country, e.g. roads and power plants.

Non-governmental organisations

Both on the international stage and within countries, non-governmental organisations (NGOs) are an increasingly important factor in discussion of development and the environment. By means of direct aid to people living in poor countries, organisations such as Oxfam can often provide services and economic assistance more cheaply than national governments. They have assumed a campaigning role on many issues connected with the poor world, and the partial success of the movement to cancel poor world debt was in no small way the result of their pressure.

In a global market of consumers, NGOs can exert pressure. In the last few years, consumer boycotts, spearheaded by NGOs, have persuaded multinational corporations to change their policies. The decision by Shell to reverse its intention to dump one of its oil rigs – Brent Spar – in the North Sea, and the consumer and farmer backlash against Monsanto for its fervent espousal of GM crops are two recent examples. NGOs were important in formulating the agenda for Rio and they have continued to make an important contribution to the sustainable development agenda. One means has been through the Commission on Sustainable Development, which was established by the United Nations to monitor progress.

Insecurity

The proponents of free markets are producing a world where insecurity is rife not only in the developing countries but also in the USA, the heartland of free markets. David Korten (1996), in his book *When Corporations Rule the World*, provides some telling illustrations of this. Only 57 per cent of the USA's non-managerial employees feel their jobs are secure. Management employees also feel insecure and Korten concludes that 'Fifty five per cent of adult Americans no longer believe that one can build a better life for oneself and one's family by working hard and playing by the rules' (Korten, 1995: 22). In other words, social cohesion is seriously damaged by a system which has elevated profit and the acquisition of money to the status of a deity. Employment is one of the pillars of a modern consumer society, a 'work and spend' society, as without it one cannot participate. The insecurity that affects American and European workers stems, in part, from the global economic system which can swiftly relocate jobs to the other side of the planet if the balance sheet dictates this. The days of one job for life and loyalty to an employer have come to an end.

Globalisation cannot be wished away. It is an economic fact with which states and individuals have to come to terms. This has led to calls for global governance – creating a set of institutions which can regulate the way in which trade is conducted in the world economy. Indeed, it can be said that this process has begun. The creation of the United Nations in 1945 spawned a series of international bodies, while the agreement between the victorious allies at Bretton Woods, New Hampshire, in 1944 created the IMF, the World Trade Organization and the World Bank. Since then, numerous international treaties have attempted to deal with social, economic and environmental problems. The relations between states, multinational corporations and their populations will be of utmost importance in the twenty-first century.

The poor world

In poor countries, the ideology of free markets is encouraging the transition to the urban industrial culture, which sucks people into cities away from the countryside and the land which has sustained their way of life for centuries. The ambition of this economic and social transformation is staggering and the impact on the planet is immense. The immersion in urban industrial life brings entry to the world market in the sense that the world's poor get that bit closer to witnessing the way of life of the rich world – they watch television, they see the tourists and their air-conditioned hotels. If they are unlucky enough, they may be forced into meeting the sexual desires of the same tourists. It is estimated that there are 500,000 child prostitutes in Thailand, Sri Lanka and the Philippines (Korten, 1996: 19). The dynamic of the contemporary industrial capitalist system is the cultivation of desire and wants, but this is utterly inappropriate in some poor world countries. There are horror stories aplenty of Western consumer products, such as baby milk powder or skin care products, being sold to poor people in developing countries who cannot afford them. What is happening is the destruction of a settled way of life lived in harmony with nature for the benefit of a culture based around the acquisition of money. The move to the city is a rupture with the past, but today that city may not be in the same country.

Economic migration across continents is made easier by the fact of globalisation. The rich world has not been able to erect adequate barriers to halt this process. Hispanics naturally gravitate to the USA and by 2050 they will form the majority of the US population (Korten, 1996). The EU states struggle to keep poor world economic migrants out of their trading bloc, but this is extremely difficult and puts immense pressure on certain countries, e.g. Spain (although it tries) cannot stop the continual flow of illegal immigrants from North Africa. To economic migration we must now add the migration of peoples caused by environmental change, which will be an increasing problem. In 1998, natural disasters uprooted more people than all the wars and conflicts that year (Monbiot, 1999). The people movement is not all one way, for the rich countries send out tourists in their millions to the poor countries. Tourism is a lucrative source of income for many poor countries, but it usually damages the local environment by responding to the needs of holiday-makers with large hotel complexes and golf courses making big demands on the local water supply. The global communications infrastructure has now enabled tourists to migrate permanently so that enclaves of Northern Europeans – mainly older people – live in southern Europe at or near Mediterranean coastal resorts. This international retirement migration is another feature of globalisation.

The impact of globalisation on the environment

The most obvious impact of globalisation is upon the environmental commons: 'those elements of the global ecosystem that are simultaneously used, experienced and shared by all and are under the effective jurisdiction or sovereignty of no one' (Held *et al.*, 1999: 378). The atmosphere, the oceans and the climate are all part of the environmental commons. The connections between the industrial way of life in the rich world with its extensive use of motor transportation and the phenomenon of global warming and climatic change are plain. The inhabitants of low-lying states are among the most obvious losers from the global climate change which is occurring. Another illustration of the connection between globalisation and the environment is transboundary pollution, which occurs, for example, when spent nuclear waste is transported from one country to another. The earth's supplies of drinkable water, grain and petroleum are put at risk by the escalating demand placed upon them by increased population in the developing world and the increasing appetites of consumer societies. The population explosion means that there will be developing conflicts over resources. The changing weather patterns look set to exacerbate this problem, turning some grain-producing areas into deserts. There is an inbuilt pressure in the world capitalist economic system to expand and innovate in order to generate more profit. This has been achieved by treating natural resources as a zero cost. The waste which is produced by this process is frequently transported around the world, very often from the rich world to the poor world.

The export of knowledge from the rich industrial countries to the poor developing countries is an example of globalisation and it can result in environmental damage when it is used to build, say, a nuclear power station (Held *et al.*, 1999: 380).

Overconsuming societies

The question of consumerism has to be at the centre of any discussion of the ways in which the world can move from its overexploitation of natural resources and climate change resulting from the urban industrial way of life. How do you persuade a population raised on consumer products that it should consume less and that, in so doing, it would enjoy a higher quality of life? Answers to this question have to be found if we are to move from the present, high-energy, resource-intensive societies of the rich world to a sustainable society. Part of the answer must surely lie in drawing public opinion into the debate on the future of consumer societies. One starting point is a projection of resource use in these societies forward to the future. Social justice requires that in a global society we consider the impact upon the environment of each country and work towards an equitable distribution of resources and energy use. People put pressure on the natural environment through their consumption of grain, fish, wood, freshwater and the pollutants they produce. When we do so, we see that the 'ecological footprint' (see Table 9.2) of each person in a consumer society is just so enormous that the level of consumption in these societies has to decline or the life-support systems of the planet will be irreversibly damaged. At present, the average North American or Japanese person consumes ten times as much of the world's resources as the average Bangladeshi person (Brown, 1998). It is not unreasonable to suppose that the industrialising developing countries will aspire to this way of life with incalculable consequences for the environment.

Consumption is central to the consideration of relations between

Table 9.2 Ecological footprints of leading industrial nations

Country	Footprint, 1993	Footprint rank
USA	8.6	1
Canada	7.2	2
Japan	7.0	3
Russian Federation	6.2	4
France	5.9	5
Germany	4.9	6
UK	4.8	7
Italy	4.7	8
World average	2.3	

Source: Mayo (1998: 2).

the developing world and the rich world. It is the consumption patterns of the rich world which are imposing insupportable demands upon the natural environment. Agenda 21 was clear about this and outlined a series of measures which would produce change in unsustainable consumption patterns. Poverty can be viewed as a part of consumption – the populations of the rich world maintain high-consumption lifestyles while over a billion people do not have enough food, have inadequate health care and lack schooling. Crucially, there will need to be a reduction in the consumer spending patterns of those living in the rich world. This will require leadership by national governments as Local Agenda 21 does not have the political weight required to effect widespread change in values and culture.

Global governance

Global governance has been creeping up on us and there is the obvious possibility that new agencies could be created which would regulate, inspect and monitor progress towards environmental sustainability.

The United Nations is generally the body associated in the popular mind with world problems and international co-operation and it usually plays a major part in crises involving conflict between states. Under the auspices of the UN over the last few decades there has been a steady accumulation of international treaties covering environmental and other important issues of concern to all nations, such as ocean pollution, Antarctica, water pollution, endangered species, toxic dumping, air pollution, conservation of wild animals, transboundary pollution and ozone depletion. The all-important Rio Earth Summit in 1992 was a United Nations initiative. This form of international co-operation as expressed in treaties is not world government as it depends for its efficacy upon the agreement of nation states. Even if a state does sign a treaty then this does not automatically mean that the country will observe the treaty. The prolonged and ultimately unsuccessful attempts of other nations to persuade the US Bush administration to change its mind and support the Kyoto agreement on global warming highlighted the difficulties.

Global co-operation is essential for responding to environmental problems. Equally, a global governance agenda would need to include social policy issues such as the regulation of labour standards (Deacon, 1998). The reform of the institutions created at Bretton Woods is high on the list of many non-governmental organisations that wish to improve social conditions and the quality of life of the poorest people of the world. There is a strong case that financial assistance should be given which would reflect environmental considerations. Fairness in trade relations between the rich and the poor world is some way off, but small initiatives prefigure what it would look like. 'Fair Trade' goods bought by consumers in the rich world – coffee, tea and other goods where most of the price goes to the producers and not to middlemen – now affects the lives of around 5 million people in the poor world (Mayo, 1998). These fairly traded products enable Western consumers to display their international and ethical orientation. Ethical trading agreements voluntarily entered into by firms have extended the concern with fairness and led to improvements in pay and conditions at work in poor countries. Consumer boycotts are another weapon which can influence trade relations between the rich and poor worlds. These initiatives do make a difference to the lives of some people in the poor world, but it is always going to be a minority. For the majority, it is international agreements between states and corporations which will have to be forged in order to protect the interests of the poorest in our world.

Environmental citizenship

Agenda 21, agreed at the Rio Summit, set out a comprehensive agenda for achieving sustainability which identified two of its priorities as the reduction of poverty and changing consumption patterns.

Green parties and green pressure groups have inserted a long-term, planetary approach into discussions of politics. This has not made them the most popular of parties with electorates used to a consumption-style politics in which politicians bid for their votes with promises of increased spending and lower taxation. The green perspectives offer a challenging and critical alternative to mainstream thinking which highlights some of the most pressing issues facing the world today. The concepts of environmental space and ecological footprint are means to demonstrate the practicalities of resource conservation, social justice for the world's poor countries today and equity for future generations. Nonetheless, this way of thinking has been making slow progress given the scale of the social and environmental problems which the world confronts. Environmental citizenship has been canvassed as a way by which ideas of environmental responsibility can grow.

Citizenship has been promoted as a unifying concept within social policy for over a century. At the beginning of the twentieth century, citizenship was used to justify the expenditure of state resources on problems of poverty and to encourage voluntary action to tackle the pressing social problems which confronted the late Victorians and Edwardians.

Shortly after the emergence of the welfare state in the 1940s, T. H. Marshall produced his famous essay on citizenship in which he argued that in the UK there has been a gradual evolution of citizenship. In the eighteenth century, the state had granted civil rights – the right to free speech and a fair trial among them – then in the course of the nineteenth and twentieth centuries the widening of the franchise ensured that political rights had been granted to the adult population. Marshall (1950) argued that after the creation of the welfare state social rights to health care, social security and education were now a reality.

Ecological citizenship builds upon the concept of social citizenship (Christoff in Doherty and de Geis, 1996). This is defined as a citizenship which seeks to extend universal principles relating to environmental rights and incorporate these in law, culture and politics. Fifty years ago, this would have appeared extremely idealistic but appears less so now for we live in an EU where there are rights which derive from European citizenship, and the European Convention on Human Rights has been incorporated into UK law.

Ecological citizenship questions the boundary between the public and the private. This will be one of the most difficult areas for many people to accept because it means that our decisions in our everyday life – such as what we do with our rubbish, how we travel, what we eat – need to be thought about in relation to their environmental consequences. In addition, ecological citizenship would assert that we recognise our obligation to animals and that in a world where we are not the only sentient creatures that we consider the impact that the human way of life is having upon animals and the rest of nature (Smith, 1998). Ecological citizenship is then seen as a way by which to transform consumer societies into societies which place a major emphasis upon the environment. It has a strong emphasis upon the obligations of the individual citizen, towards non-humans, future generations and foreign peoples who are affected by our actions. As Barry (1999: 231) writes, 'citizenship, as viewed by green democratic theory, emphasizes the duty of citizens to take responsibility for their actions and choices – the obligation to "do one's bit" in the collective enterprise of achieving sustainability'. In this sense, states can do a great deal, but they need individuals to carry out their responsibilities in such areas as the conservation of energy, recycling and environmentally aware consumption.

It is not possible to be sanguine about the power of such ideas to change perceptions as, in the UK and other rich societies, there is now no agreed version of public morality; instead, there is a host of competing ideas about morality, and related to this there is a strong mood among the population that they do not want to be told how to behave. This derives from decades of consumerism during which rights have been stressed and obligations downplayed. Consumer societies may lose their appeal in a world where global warming has produced severe weather patterns which have disrupted nation states and the world economy to such an extent that ecological citizenship is the only realistic option.

Key points

- Globalisation is distinguished by the removal of time and space barriers via information technology and the doctrine of free markets.
- The environment and poor countries are being exploited by this global economic system.
- Global governance and global citizenship are ways of responding to the need for sustainable development.

Guide to further reading

Deacon, B. (1998) *Global Social Policy*, London: Sage. Discussion of the impact of globalisation on social policy.

Gorringe, T. (1999) *Fair Shares: Ethics and the Global Economy*, London: Thames and Hudson. Argument that the obsession with money has led to a deterioration in moral values which can be remedied via the adoption of green ethics.

Gray, J. (1998) *False Dawn: the Delusions of Global Capitalism*, London: Granta Books. Fierce polemic against the advocates of free markets.

Held, D., McGrew, A., Goldblatt, D. and Perraton, J. (1999) *Global Transformations*, Cambridge: Polity Press. Undoubtedly the most authoritative account of contemporary globalisation.

Hertz, N. (2001) *The Silent Takeover: Global Capitalism and the Death of Democracy*, London: William Heinemann. Description of the ways in which corporate business is assuming numerous functions previously perfomed by the state.

Klein, N. (2000) *No Logo*, London: Flamingo. Compelling explanation of the power of consumerism and the emerging global resistance.

Web sites

Corporate Watch (www.corpwatch.org).
Fair Trade Foundation (www.fairtrade.org.uk).
Oxfam (www.oxfam.org).
United Nations (www.un.org).
World Bank (www.worldbank.org).
World Trade Organization (www.wto.org).

Bibliography

Agyeman, J. and Evans, B. (1996) 'Sustainability and democracy, community participation in Local Agenda 21', *Local Government Policy Making* 22 (2), 35–40.

Atkinson, A.B. (1996) 'The case for a participation income', *Political Quarterly* 67, 67–70.

Audit Commission (1997) *It's a Small World: Local Government's Role as a Steward of the Environment*, London: HMSO.

Bahro, R. (1982) *Socialism and Survival*, London: Heretic Books.

Bahro, R. (1986) *Building the Green Movement*, London: Heretic Books.

Barnes, P.M. and Barnes, I.G. (1999) *Environmental Policy in the European Union*, Cheltenham: Edward Elgar.

Barnes, H., North, P. and Walker, P. (1996) *LETS on Low Income*, London: New Economics Foundation.

Barry, J. (1999) *Rethinking Green Politics*, London: Sage.

Bateman, D. (1995) 'Local Agenda 21', *Local Government Policy Making* 22 (2), 16–20.

Baumann, Z. (1994) *Alone Again: Ethics after Certainty*, London: Demos.

Bell, S. and Morse, S. (1999) *Sustainability Indicators: Measuring the Immeasurable*, London: Earthscan.

Bhatti, M., Brooke, J. and Gibson, M. (eds) (1994) *Housing and the Environment: a New Agenda*, Coventry: Chartered Institute of Housing.

Blowers, A. (ed.) (1993) *Planning for a Sustainable Environment*, London: Earthscan.

Boardman, B. (1998) *Rural Transport Policy and Equity*, London: CPRE Countryside Commission and Rural Development Commission.

Bocock, R. (1993) *Consumption,* London: Routledge.

Boseley, S. (1999) 'Health drive as obesity soars', *Guardian* 1 April, 9.

Bowring, F. (1998) 'LETS, an eco-socialist initiative?', *New Left Review* November–December (232): 91–111.

Boyle, D. (1999) *Funny Money*, London: HarperCollins.

Bramwell, A. (1989) *Ecology in the 20th Century: A History*, London: Yale University Press.

Brandt, B. (1995) *Whole Life Economics: Revaluing Daily Life*, Philadelphia: New Society Publishers.

Breheny, M.J. (ed.) (1992) *Sustainable Development and Urban Form*, London: Pion.

Breheny, M. (1999) 'The People – where will they work?', *Town and Country Planning*, December.

British Medical Association (1998) *Health and Environmental Impact Assessment*, London: Earthscan.

Brown, P. (1998) 'Road accidents set to be world's biggest killer', *Guardian* 24 June, 14.

Brown, L.R. and Flavin, C. (1999) *State of the World*, London: Earthscan.

Brown, L.R., Renner, M. and Flavin, C. (1998) *Vital Signs 1998–1999*, London: Earthscan.

CAG Consultants (1998) *Perceptions of National Barriers to Local Sustainability*, London: CAG.

Cahn, E. (1986) *Service Credits: a New Currency for the Welfare State*, London: London School of Economics.

Carley, M. and Kirk, K. (1998) *Sustainable by 2020?*, Bristol: The Policy Press and the Joseph Rowntree Foundation.

Carley, M. and Spapens, P. (1998) *Sharing the World: Sustainable Living and Global Equity in the 21st Century*, London: Earthscan.

Carlson, J. (1997) 'A feminist assessment of BI: problems and prospects', unpublished paper, Social Policy Association Annual Conference.

Carson, R. (1962) *Silent Spring*, New York: Fawcett Crest Pepper.

Central Statistical Office (1995) *Social Trends*, London: HMSO.

Christie, I. (1996) 'A green light for local power', *Demos* 9.

Clement, B. (1996) 'No rest for the British', *Independent* 4 August, 17.

Conaty, P. and Mayo, E. (1997) *A Commitment to People and Place: the Case for Community Development Credit Unions*, London: New Economics Foundation.

Connelly, J. and Smith, G. (1999) *Politics and the Environment, from Theory to Practice*, London: Routledge.

Consumers' Association (1999) 'UK's inefficient homes use record amounts', press release.

Conway, G. (1997) *The Doubly Green Revolution*, London: Penguin Books.

Cooper, G (1995a) 'School dinners "can damage your health"' *Independent* 3 November, 7.

Cooper, G. (1995b) 'Feeding an appetite for restaurants' *Independent* 15 November, 4.

Crombie, H. (1995) *Sustainable Development and Health*, Birmingham: Public Health Alliance.

Dalal-Clayton, B. (1996) *Getting to Grips with Green Plans*, London: Earthscan.

Daly, H.E. (ed.) (1980) *Economics, Ecology, Ethics: Essays Towards a Steady-state Economy*, San Francisco: W. H. Freeman.

Dauncey, G. (1988) *After the Crash: The Emergence of the Rainbow Economy*, Basingstoke: Green Print.

Davies, J.K. and Kelly, M. (eds) (1993) *Healthy Cities: Research and Practice*, London: Routledge.

Deacon, B. (1998) *Global Social Policy*, London: Sage.

Demos (1994) 'Special employment issue', *Demos Quarterly* 2.

Department of the Environment (1990) *This Common Inheritance*, Cm. 1200, London: HMSO.

Department of the Environment (1994) *Sustainable Development: the UK Strategy*, London: HMSO.

Department of the Environment (1995) *Rural England: a Nation Committed to a Living Countryside*, Cm. 3016, London: HMSO.

Department of the Environment, Transport and the Regions (1998a) *Sustainability Counts*, London: DETR.

Department of the Environment, Transport and the Regions (1998b) *A New Deal for Transport, Better for Everyone*, Cm. 3950, London: HMSO.

Department of the Environment, Transport and the Regions (1998c) *Sustainable Local Communities for the 21st Century – Why and How to Prepare an Effective Local Agenda 21 Strategy*, London: DETR.

Department of the Environment, Transport and the Regions (1998d) *Modern Local Government: in Touch with the People*, Cm. 4014, London: HMSO.

Department of the Environment, Transport and the Regions (1999a) *A Better Quality of Life: a Strategy for Sustainable Development in the UK*, Cm. 4345, London: DETR.

Department of the Environment, Transport and the Regions (1999b) *Fuel Poverty: The New HEES*, London: DETR.

Department of the Environment, Transport and the Regions (2000) *The 10 Year Plan*, London: HMSO.

Department of Health (1976) *Prevention and Health: Everybody's Business*, London: HMSO.

Department of Health (1995) 'National Diet and Nutrition Survey of Pre-School Children', press release, 22 March 1995, 95/149.

Department of Health (1996) *The United Kingdom National Environmental Health Action Plan*, Cm. 3323, London: HMSO.

Department of Health (1998a) *Our Healthier Nation, a Contract for Health*, Cm. 3852, London: HMSO.

Department of Health (1998b) *Independent Enquiry into Inequalities in Health (Acheson Report)*, London: HMSO.

Department of Health (1999) *Saving Lives: Our Healthier Nation*, Cm. 4386, London: HMSO.

Department of Health Committee on the Medical Effects of Air Pollutants (1997) *Handbook on Air Pollution and Health*, London: HMSO.

Devall, B. (1990) *Simple in Means, Rich in Ends: Practising Deep Ecology*, London: Green Print.

Dobson, A. (ed.) (1999) *Fairness and Futurity: Essays on Environmental Sustainability and Social Justice*, Oxford: Oxford University Press.

Dobson, A. (2000) *Green Political Thought*, 3rd edn, London: Routledge.

Dodds, F. (ed.) (1997) *The Way Forward: Beyond Agenda 21*, London: Earthscan.

Doherty, B. and de Geis, M. (1996) *Democracy and Green Political Thought: Sustainable Rights and Citizenship*, London: Routledge.

Douthwaite, R. (1996) *Short Circuit: Strengthening Local Economics for Security in an Unstable World*, Dartington: Green Books.

Draper, P. (ed.) (1991) *Health Through Public Policy: the Greening of Public Health*, London: Green Print.

Dryzek, J.S. (1997) *The Politics of the Earth: Environmental Discourses*, Oxford: Oxford University Press.

Eckersley, R. (1992) *Environmentalism and Political Theory: Towards an Ecocentric Approach*, London: UCL Press.

Elkin, T., McLaren, D. and Hillman, M. (1991) *Reviving the City: Towards Sustainable Urban Development Environment*, London: Friends of the Earth/Policy Studies Institute.

Elliott, L. and Brittain, V. (1998) 'The rich and poor grow further apart', *Guardian* 9 September, 18.

Etzioni, A. (1995) *The Spirit of Community*, London: Fontana Press.

European Commission (1993) *Towards Sustainability: The Fifth EC Environmental Action Programme*, Brussels: Directorate General XI.

European Commission (1996) *European Sustainable Cities – Report of the Expert Group on the Urban Environment DG X1*, Brussels: European Commission.

European Commission (2001) 'Commission organises "name and shame" seminar on city sewage', press release, 19 March, Brussels: European Commission.

European Federation of Road Traffic Victims (1997) *Impact of Road Death and Injury*, Geneva: ERTV.

Fairlie, S. (1996) *Low Impact Development*, Charlbury: Jon Carpenter.

Festing, H. (1998a) *Farmers' Markets, an American Success Story*, Bristol: Ecologic.

Festing, H. (1998b) 'So you want to start a Farmers' Market?', *Town and Country Planning* July, 216–19.

Fifth Report House of Commons Select Committee *The Future for Allotments*, London: HMSO.

Fitzpatrick, T. (1999) *Freedom and Security: an Introduction to the Basic Income Debate*, London: Macmillan.

Fodor, M., Speeden, S. and Whittaker, S. (1995) 'Fostering a Corporate Approach to Local Agenda 21 – using Performance Review', *Local Government Policy Making* 22: 21–27.

Frank, R.H. (1999) *Luxury Fever: Money and Happiness in an Age of Excess*, Princeton, NJ: Princeton University Press.

Freeman, C., Littlewood, S. and Whitney, D. (1996) 'Local government and emerging models of participation in the Local Agenda 21 process', *Journal of Environmental Planning and Management* 39, 65–78.

Friends of the Earth (1998a) *Perceptions of National Barriers to Local Sustainability*, London: CAG Consultants.

Friends of the Earth (1998b) *Water Pollution*, London: Friends of the Earth.

Friends of the Earth (1999) 'Pollution injustice', press briefing.

Fyfe, G. (ed.) (1994) *Poor and Paying for It*, London: HMSO.

Garner, R. (2000) *Environmental Politics*, 2nd edn, Basingstoke: Macmillan.

Garreau, J. (1992) *Edge City: Life on the New Frontier*, New York: Doubleday.

Gaskin, K. (1998) 'Vanishing volunteers, are young people losing interest in volunteering?', *Voluntary Action* 1 (winter), 1, 33–43.

George, V. and Page, R. (eds) (1995) *Modern Thinkers on Welfare*, London: Harvester Wheatsheaf.

Girardet, H. (1996a) *The Gaia Atlas of Cities*, London: Gaia.

Girardet, H. (1996b) *Gaia Atlas of Planet Management*, London: Gaia.

Girardet, H (1999) *Creating Sustainable Cities*, Dartington: Green Books.

Gorz, A. (1989) *Critique of Economic Reason*, London: Verso.

Gray, J. (1993) *Beyond the New Right: Markets, Government and the Common Environment*, London: Routledge.

Gray, J. (1998) *False Dawn, the Delusions of Global Capitalism*, London: Granta Books.

Hakim, C. (1996) *Key Issues in Women's Work*, London: Athlone Press.

Hall, P. and Ward, C. (1998) *Sociable Cities: the Legacy of Ebenezer Howard*, Chichester: John Wiley.

Hamer, L. (1999) *Making T.H.E links, Integrating Sustainable Transport, Health and Environmental Policies: A Guide for Local Authorities and Health Authorities*, London: Health Education Authority.

Handy, C. (1984) *The Future of Work*, Oxford: Blackwell.

Hardin, G. (1968) 'The Tragedy of the Commons', in Dryzek, J.S. and Schlosberg, D. (eds) (1998) *Debating the Earth: The Environmental Politics Reader*, Oxford: Oxford University Press.

Harding, L. (1997)'Britons binge on sweets', *Guardian* 8 January, 7.

Harper, C. (1996) *Environment and Society: Human Perspectives on Environmental Issues*, New Jersey: Prentice Hall.

Health Education Authority (1998) *Transport and Health*, London: Health Education Authority.

Held, D., McGrew, A., Goldblatt, D. and Perraton, J. (1999) *Global Transformations*, Cambridge: Polity Press.

Henderson, H. (1999) *Beyond Globalisation: Shaping a Sustainable Global Economy*, Connecticut: Kumarian Press.

Henson, S. and Gregory, S. (eds) (1994) *The Politics of Food,* occasional paper no. 2, Reading: University of Reading Department of Agricultural Economics and Management.

Higgins, J. (1978) *The Poverty Business Britain and America*, Oxford: Blackwell.

Himmelfarb, G. (1984) *The Idea of Poverty: England in the Early Industrial Age*, London: Faber and Faber.

Hirsch, F. (1977) *Social Limits to Growth*, London: Routledge.

Hochschild, A. (1997) *The Time Bind: When Work Becomes Home and Home Becomes Work*, New York: Metropolitan Books, Henry Holt.

Howard, E. (1902) *Garden Cities of Tomorrow*, London: Faber and Faber.

House of Commons (2001) *Organic Farming: House of Commons Agriculture Committee Second Report,* Vol. 1, HC 149-1, London: HMSO.

House of Commons Select Committee on the Environment, Transport and the Regions (1998) The Future for Allotments, HC 560-1, London: HMSO.

Huby, M. (1998) *Social Policy and the Environment*, Buckingham: Open University Press.

Huby, M. (2000) 'Food and the environment', in May, M., Brunsden, E. and Page, R. (eds) *Social Problems in Social Policy*, Oxford: Blackwell.

Hudson, H., Newby, L., Hutchinson, N. with Harding, L. (1999) *Making 'LETS' Work in Low Income Areas*, London: Forum for the Future.

Hunt, L. (1996) 'Obesity crisis needs medical answer', *Independent* 13 March, 7.

Instituto del Tercer Mundo (1997) *The World Guide 1997/98*, Oxford, New Internationalist Publications.

Jacobs, M. (ed.) (1997) *Greening the Millennium? The New Politics of the Environment*, Oxford: Blackwell.

Jacobs, M. (1999) *Environmental Modernisation*, London: Fabian Society.

James, O. (1997) *Britain on the Couch*, London: Century.

Jenks, M., Burton, E. and Williams, K. (1996) *The Compact City: a Sustainable Urban Form?*, London: E and FN Spon.

Jones, L. and Siddell, M. (eds) (1997) *The Challenge of Promoting Health*, London: Macmillan/Open University Press.

Katz, P. (ed.) (1994) *New Urbanism: Towards an Architecture of Community*, New York: McGraw Hill.

Kocher, P. and Williamson, V. (1996) *Local Agenda 21: Introducing a Dialogue with Local People on Environmental Policy*, Brighton: University of Brighton Health and Social Policy Research Centre.

Korten, D. (1996) *When Corporations Rule the World*, London: Earthscan.

Labour Party (1997) *New Labour: Because Britain Deserves Better*, London: Labour Party.

Lambert, R. (1964) *Nutrition in Britain 1950–1960*, London: G. Bell.

Lancashire County Council (1997) *Lancashire's Green Audit 2: A Sustainability Report*, Preston: Lancashire County Council.

Lang, P. (1994) *LETS Work: Rebuilding the Local Economy*, Bristol: Grover Books.

Lang, T. (1997) *Food Policy for the 21st Century: Can it be Both Radical and Reasonable?*, London: Thames Valley University, Centre for Food Policy.

Lang, T. and Hines, C. (1993) *The New Protectionism: Protecting the Future Against Free Trade*, London: Earthscan.

Lang, T., Caraher, M., Dixon, P. and Carr-Hill, R. (1999) *Cooking Skills and Health*, London: Health Education Authority.

Lasch, C. (1995) *The Revolt of the Elites and the Betrayal of Democracy*, New York: W.W. Norton.

Lawrence, J.G. (1998) 'Getting the Future that You Want: The Role of Sustainability Indicators', in Warburton, D. (ed.) *Community and Sustainable Development: Participation in the Future*, London: Earthscan.

Lean, G. (1998) 'It's the poor that do the suffering', *New Statesman* 16 October, 10–11.

Leather, S. (1996) *The Making of Modern Malnutrition, an Overview of Food Poverty in the UK*, London: Caroline Walker Trust.

Local Government Management Board (1996) *New Profession for a New Agenda? Environmental Coordinators in Local Government*, Luton: LGMB, London: Routledge.

MacGillivray, A. (1998) 'Turning the Sustainability Corner: How to Indicate Right', in Warburton, D. (ed.) *Community and Sustainable Development: Participation in the Future*, London: Earthscan.

McKibben, B. (1990) *The End of Nature*, Harmondsworth: Penguin.

McLaren, D., Bullock, S. and Yousuf, N. (1998) *Tomorrow's World: Britain's Share in a Sustainable Future*, London: Earthscan.

McMichael, A.J. (1993) *Planetary Overload, Global Environmental Change and the Health of the Human Species*, Cambridge: Cambridge University Press.

Macnaghten, P. and Urry, J. (1998) *Contested Natures*, London: Sage.

Maddison, D., Pearce, D., Johansson, O., Catlthrop, E., Litman, T. and Verhoef, E. (1996) *The True Costs of Road Transport*, London: Kogan Page.

Malthus, T.R. (1970) *An Essay on the Principle of Population*, Harmondsworth: Penguin (first published in 1798).

Marine Conservation Society (2001) 'Sewage pollution', http://www.mcsuk.org/marineworld/sewage_html.

Marshall, T.H. (1950, reprinted 1992) *Citizenship and Social Class*, London: Pluto Press.

Mayo, E. (1998) *Making New Economics: Proposals for the G8 1998 Summits*, London: New Economics Foundation.

Mayo, E., Fisher, T., Conaty, P., Doling, J. and Mullineux, A. (1998) *Small is Bankable: Community Reinvestment in the UK*, York: Joseph Rowntree Foundation in association with New Economics Foundation.

Meadows, D.H., Meadows, D.L. and Randers, J. (1972) *The Limits to Growth*, New York: Universe Books.

Meikle, J. (1998) 'Food poisoning', *Guardian* 14 January, 15.

Meikle, J. (1999) 'Children's diet healthier in 1950 than today', *Guardian* 30 November, 4.

Meikle, J. (2000) 'Scientists find new BSE links', *Guardian* 29 August, 1.

Mellor, M. (1997) *Feminism and Ecology*, Cambridge: Polity Press.

Miles, S. (1998) *Consumerism as a Way of Life*, London: Sage.

Miller, S. (1997) 'Television shatters dinner chatter', *Guardian* 29 September, 5.

Ministry of Agriculture (1998) *The Food Standards Agency: a Force for Change*, London: HMSO.

Mintel (1997) *Food Retailing: Retail Intelligence*, March, 1–30.

Monbiot, G. (1999) 'Apocalypse Now', *Guardian* 29 July, 20.

Morris, J. (1998) 'Coming in from the cold', *Town and Country Planning* January/February.

Morris, W. (1890) *News from Nowhere*, Boston: Roberts Brothers.

Mulgan, G. (1997) *Connexity*, London: Chatto and Windus.

Murcott, A. (ed.) (1998) *'The Nation's Diet': the Social Science of Food Choice*, Harlow: Addison, Wesley Longman.

Office for National Statistics (1997) *Regional Trends 32*, 1997 edition, London: HMSO.

O'Hara, M. (2000) 'Italian food boom reaches new heights', *Guardian* 30 August, 23.

O'Riordan, T. and Voisey, H. (eds) (1998) *The Transition to Sustainability: The Politics of Agenda 21 in Europe*, London: Earthscan.

Pearce, D. (1989) *Blueprint for a Green Economy*, London: Earthscan.

Pepper, D. (1993) *Eco-socialism: from Deep Ecology to Social Justice*, London: Routledge.

Pepper, D. (1996) *Modern Environmentalism: an Introduction*, London: Routledge.

Percy, S. (1998) 'Real Progress or Optimistic Hype?', *Town and Country Planning* January/February, 11–13.

Phillimore, P. and Moffat, S. (1999) 'Narratives of insecurity in Teesside', in Vail, J., Wheelock, J. and Hill, M. (eds) *Insecure Times*, London: Routledge.

Porritt, J. (1984) *Seeing Green*, Oxford: Basil Blackwell.

Porritt, J. (2000) *Playing Safe, Science and the Environment*, London: Thames and Hudson.

Potter, S. (1997) *Vital Travel Statistics*, London: Landor.

Power, A. and Mumford, K. (1999) *'The Slow Death of Great Cities?'*, York: Joseph Rowntree Foundation.

Raven, H., Lang, T. and Dumonteil, C. (1995) *Off our Trolleys? Food Retailing and the Hypermarket Economy*, London: Institute of Public Policy Research.

Reeves, R. (2000) 'All change in the workplace', *Observer* 30 January, 18.

Riches, G. (ed.) (1997) *First World Hunger, Food Security and Welfare Politics*, London: Macmillan.

Robertson, J. (1996) 'Towards a new social compact, Citizen's Income and Radical Tax Reform', *Political Quarterly* 67, 54–8.

Robertson, J. (1998) *Transforming Economic Life, a Millennial Challenge*, Dartington: Green Books.

Rosenbaum, M. (1993) *Children and the Environment*, London: National Children's Bureau.

Rowell, A., Holman, H. and Sohi, S. (1992) *Populations at Risk from Ambient Air Pollution in England*, London: Greenpeace.

Royal Commission on Environmental Pollution (1997) *Twentieth Report, Transport and the Environment – Developments since 1994*, London: HMSO.

Rudlin, D. (1998) *Tomorrow: a Peaceful Path to Urban Reform*, London: Friends of the Earth.

Rudlin, D. and Falk, N. (1999) *Building the 21st Century Home*, Oxford: Architectural Press.

Rugg, J. and Jones, A. (1999) *Getting a Job, Finding a Home, Rural Youth Transitions*, York: Joseph Rowntree foundation.

Sachs, W., Loske, R. and Linz, M. (1998) *Greening the North*, London: Zed Books.

Selman, P. (1996) *Local Sustainability*, London: Paul Chapman.

Senaur, R., Asp, E. and Kinsey, J. (1991) *Food Trends and the Changing Consumer*, Minnesota: Eagan Press.

Sherlock, H. (1991) *Cities are Good for Us*, London: Paladin.

Shucksmith, M. (2000) *Exclusive Countryside? Social Inclusion and Regeneration in Rural Areas*, York: Joseph Rowntree Foundation.

Smith, M.J. (1998) *Ecologism, Towards Ecological Citizenship*, Buckingham: Open University Press.

Smith, M., Whitelegg, J. and Williams, N. (1998) *Greening the Built Environment*, London: Earthscan.

Stevenson, J. (1984) *British Society 1914–45*, Harmondsworth: Penguin Books.

Stott, M. (1998) 'Don't lose the plot', *Town and Country Planning* March, 5.

Tansey, G. and Worsley, T. (1995) *The Food System: a Guide*, London: Earthscan.

Taylor, M. (1998) *Unleashing the Potential*, York: Joseph Rowntree Foundation.

Tickell, O. (1998) 'Road accidents kill or disable more people than TB, war or HiV', *Guardian* 24 June, 4.

Tindale, S. (1996) 'Procrastination, precaution and the global gamble', in Franklin, J. (ed.) *The Politics of Risk Society*, Cambridge: Polity Press.

Treanor, J. (1999) 'Computer age widens deficit', *Guardian* 7 July, 24.

Turok, I. (1999) 'Squeezing Surrey to sustain Sunderland?', *Town and Country Planning* September, 268–9.

United Nations (1992) *Report of the United Nations Conference on Environment and Development, Agenda 21, Rio de Janeiro, 3–14 June 1992*, Geneva: United Nations.

United Nations Development Programme (1999) *Human Development Report 1999*, Oxford: Oxford University Press.

Urban Task Force (1999) *Towards an Urban Renaissance*, London: E and FN Spon.

Vail, J., Wheelock, J. and Hill, M. (1999) *Insecure Times: Living with Insecurity in Contemporary Society*, London: Routledge.

Vidal, J. (1999) 'First among equals', *Guardian* 3 March, 4.

Von Weizsacker, E., Lovins, A.B. and Lovins, L.H. (1997) *Factor Four: Doubling Wealth, Halving Resource Use*, London: Earthscan.

Wall, A. and Owen, B. (1999) *Health Policy*, Eastbourne: Gildredge Press.

Walters, J. (2001) 'War on the car sparks driver rage', *The Observer* 26 August, 1.

Warburton, D. (ed.) (1998) *Community and Sustainable Development: Participation in the Future*, London: Earthscan.

Ward, S. (1993) *Thinking Global, Acting Local? Local Authorities and their Environmental Plans*, Bristol: University of the West of England.

Webster, C. (1990) *The Victorian Public Health Legacy: A Challenge to the Future*, Birmingham: Institution of Environmental Health Officers/The Public Health Alliance.

Wheelock, J. and Vail, J. (1998) *Work and Idleness, the Political Economy of Full Employment*, London: Kluwer Academic Publishers.

Wilkinson, R.G. (1996) *Unhealthy Societies: the Afflictions of Inequality*, London: Routledge.

Wilkinson, H. and Howard, M. (1997) *Tomorrow's Women*, London: Demos.

Wilson, J. (1999) 'Green and pleasant land "at risk" as meadows disappear', *Guardian* 15 March, 4.

World Commission on Environment and Development (Brundtland Report) (1987) *Our Common Future*, Oxford: Oxford University Press.

Worpole, K. (1992) *Towns for People: Transforming Urban Life*, Buckingham: Open University Press.

Young, S.C. (1997) 'Local Agenda 21, the renewal of local democracy?', in Jacobs, M. (ed.) *Greening the Millennium? The New Politics of the Environment*, Oxford: Blackwell.

Young, B. (1988) 'Prize Guize', *Guardian*, 11 March, 4.

Index

affluence 8
Agenda 21 20, 30–1; and joined-up government 33
air pollution 14, 71–5
allotments 50, 119

Bahro, Rudolf 57–8
banks, 142–3
Blair, Tony 25
Bookchin, Murray 59–60
Boyd Orr, Sir John 120
Brundtland Report 2, 3, 17, 43
BSE (bovine spongiform encephalopathy) 125–6

Cahn, Edgar 149
capacity building 36
car dependence 26, 96; and food shopping 121; geography of employment 137; pollution 73–5; positional good 10; in rural areas 101
Carson, Rachel 116
children: and day care 90; and diet 123–4; and employment 138; parental employment 141, 151
Citizen's Income 143–5
citizenship 165; ecological citizenship 164–6
CJD (Creutzfeldt–Jakob disease) 126
climate change 65–6, 113, 161
Club of Rome Report 1971 11
Commission on Sustainable Development 29
commodification 139
Common Agricultural Policy 115, 129–30

consumerism 16, 48–9, 161–3, 166
consumer society 8–10
consumption 16–17
convenience food 119, 122
cooking 118–19
Corporate Watch 167
Council for the Protection of Rural England 112
country life 99
Countryside Agency 112
Credit Unions 143
Currie, Edwina 126

Darwin, Charles 51
DEFRA (Department of the Environment, Food and Rural Affairs) 29, 129, 132
DETR (Department of the Environment, Transport and the Regions) 25
DTLR (Department of Transport, Local Government and the Regions) 46

Earth Summit: Johannesburg 46; New York 20, 25; Rio 19, 30, 62, 163;
ecocentric 53
eco-feminism 60
ecology 82
ecological footprint 13, 110, 162
ecological modernisation 21, 62–3
economic growth 10–11
eco-socialism 56–9
employment: and housing 103–4; and industrialisation 134–6; in the UK 136–7; women's employment 136

energy 105–6
Environment Agency 88
environmental citizenship 164–6
environmental injustice 14, 73
environmental policy 31–2
environmental risk 70–1
environmental space 12, 164–5
environmental taxation 15, 28
European Union environmental
    policy 23–5; Fifth Environmental
    Action Programme 23, 24

Fair Trade 164
Fair Trade Foundation 167
farmers' markets 117–18; National
    Association of Farmers' Markets
    132
farming 116
financial exclusion 142–3
food: children's diet 123–5;
    convenience 118–19, 122; cooking
    118–19; food deserts 117, 119;
    genetically modified food 126,
    128; organic food 117; food miles
    115, 118, 125; packaging 125;
    food poverty 120–1; food security
    128
Food Commission 132
food policy: and allotments 119;
    damage to eco-sphere 114–15;
    farmers' markets 117–18; and
    farming 116; government policy
    128–30; Ministry of Food 129;
    and obesity 122, 124–5; and poor
    diet 121–5; and retailing 117;
    school meals 124
Food Standards Agency 130–1, 132
Frank, Robert H. 89–90
free markets 157–8; 159
Friends of the Earth 52, 84, 102;
    survey of Local Agenda 21 42–3;
    survey of industrial pollution 72–3
fuel poverty 107–8

garden cities 95–6, 110
globalisation 154–8; and the
    environment 161

global governance 159, 163
global warming 25, 65, 104, 153,
    154, 161
Gorz, André 58–9
Gray, John 61
green belt 90
green conservatism 61
green ideologies 47–64
Greenpeace 52
greens: dark greens 53–6; green
    parties 52–3; green conservatives
    61; *see also* eco-socialism; eco-
    feminism

Haeckel, Ernest 52
Hardin, Garret 53–5
Health Action Zones 87–8
Health Improvement Programmes
    33, 87
Health of the Nation 85
health promotion 84
healthy cities 82–3, 91
Hirsch, Fred 10
Home Energy Conservation Act 1995
    106
Home Energy Efficiency Scheme
    106
household skills 139
housing: and employment 103–4;
    and energy 105–6; and fuel
    poverty 107–8
Howard, Ebenezer 95–6, 110, 112

IMF (International Monetary Fund)
    157–8industrialisation: critics of
    50; and employment 134–5; and
    the environment 3–4; and health
    67–8; and housing 93–4; and
    population 51
inequality 14
insecurity 158–9

Jacobs, Michael 2
Johannesburg Earth Summit 46
joined-up government: in central
    government 86; in local
    authorities 33

Kerala 13
Korten, David 159

Lancashire County Council 39
Lawrence, J. Gary 40–2
Limits to Growth report 8, 11
Local Agenda 21 30–46; and
    capacity building 36; and
    community strategy 46; and
    participation 35–7; and
    partnership 37; and poverty 38–40
local authorities 31–45
Local Exchange Trading Systems
    (LETS) 145–9

Macmillan, Harold 8
Major, John 32, 33
Malthus, Rev. Thomas 51
Marshall, T.H. 165
migration: economic migration 160;
    international retirement migration
    160; in the poor world 69
Ministry of Agriculture 129, 131
Morris, William 50, 57

noise 77, 80
non-governmental organisations 158

obesity 122
Our Healthier Nation 85–7, 89
Oxfam 167
own work 151

participation: community
    participation 36; in local
    government 35–6
Pearce, David 21
pollution: air pollution 71–5; indoor
    pollutants 81–2; noise pollution
    77, 80; transport pollution 73–5;
    water pollution 80–1
population 51; growth in rural areas
    99
poverty 163
public health 67–9

Quality of Life 14–16; 26–8

risk 70–1
road accidents 75–7
Robertson, James 144–5
Rogers, Richard 103
romantic critiques 50
rural inequality 100
rurbanisation 99
Ruskin, John 50

safety 98–9
school meals 124
shopping 9
smoking 81–2, 84, 121
social capital 36–7, 89
social citizenship 165
social ecology 59–60
social economy 141–2
social justice 6–7, 162, 165
social policy 2–3, 16–17, 18, 134
suburbs 94–6
sustainability 1–2, 6; and housing
    103–4
sustainability indicators 35, 40–2
sustainable cities 109–11
sustainable development 2, 5, 19–29;
    and Conservative governments
    21–2, 28; and European Union
    23–5; and New Labour
    government 25–6, 28–9

Thatcher, Margaret 21, 32–3, 61
time deprivation 138, 140–1
time dollars 149–50
tourism 160
Town and Country Planning
    Association 112
transport 25–6, 94–5; and health 75–
    9, 105; and pollution 73–5; and
    rural inequality 101; and
    sustainability indicators 40
travel to work 97–8

United Nations 159, 163, 167
Urban Development Corporations 97
urbanisation: opposition to 50; global
    93; and health 69; in the UK 93–4
urban policy 96–9
urban renaissance 102–3

water: consumption 108–9;
    contamination 14; metering 81;
    sewage 81
Welfare State 3
work: and consumer society 135,
    151; and industrialisation 134; job
    addiction 141; public work 137;
    redistribution of work 150–1; and
    social policy 134; in the UK 136–
    7; voluntary work 139–40; work
poor 138; work rich 138;
    work and spend society 135,
    140
World Bank 157–8, 167
World Commission on Environment
    and Development *see* Brundtland
    Report
World Health Organization 70–1, 72,
    76, 77, 82–3, 91
World Trade Organization 157, 167

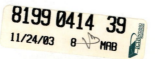